# Esophageal Surgery - Current Principles and Advances

*Edited by Andrea Sanna*

Published in London, United Kingdom

Esophageal Surgery - Current Principles and Advances
http://dx.doi.org/10.5772/intechopen.102237
Edited by Andrea Sanna

Contributors
Gad Marom, Ronit Brodie, Yoav Mintz, José Luis Braga de Aquino, Vânia Aparecida Leandro-Merhi, Jihwan Ko, Robert F. Cubas, Maria Carolina Jimenez, Jose M. Martinez, Srijan Shukla, Subramanyesh Rao Thammineedi, Sujit Chyau Patnaik, Nusrath Syed, Ajesh Raj Saksena, Pratap Reddy Ramalingam, Andrea Sanna, Enrico Piva



First published in London, United Kingdom, 2023 by IntechOpen
IntechOpen is the global imprint of INTECHOPEN LIMITED, registered in England and Wales, registration number: 11086078, 5 Princes Gate Court, London, SW7 2QJ, United Kingdom

British Library Cataloguing-in-Publication Data
A catalogue record for this book is available from the British Library

Additional hard and PDF copies can be obtained from orders@intechopen.com

Esophageal Surgery - Current Principles and Advances
Edited by Andrea Sanna
p. cm.
Print ISBN 978-1-80356-797-6
Online ISBN 978-1-80356-798-3
eBook (PDF) ISBN 978-1-80356-799-0

# Meet the editor

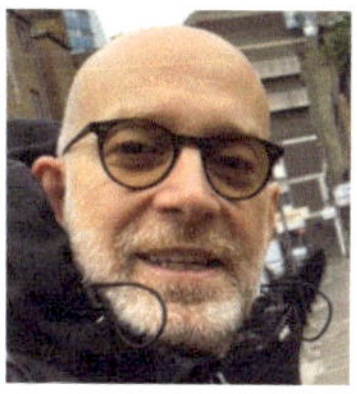

Andrea Sanna, MD, is a highly qualified surgeon and the head of the General Surgery Unit at Saint Mary of Angels Hospital in Adria, Italy. He completed his general surgery degree at Ferrara University and has since focused on several clinical interests, including advanced minimally invasive surgery, abdominal wall reconstruction, endocrine surgery, and emergency surgery. He specializes in laparoscopic colon and gastric cancer surgeries, laparoscopic and endoscopic primary and incisional abdominal wall reconstruction, minimally invasive thyroidectomy and parathyroidectomy, and the Desarda's groin hernia repair technique. Dr. Sanna has contributed several articles and book chapters on general surgery and is an active member of various surgical associations.

# Contents

# Preface

*Esophageal Surgery - Current Principles and Advances* is a collection of chapters concerning technology innovation in medical practice. It covers a wide range of applications of esophageal surgery in fields of medicine such as radiology, gastroenterology and surgery.

This book is written for healthcare professionals wishing to understand the principles and applications of new technology in esophageal surgery. The material is accessible to anyone, regardless of technical skills. It is suitable as a textbook for undergraduate and postgraduate clinical training. I hope that other experts will be encouraged to contribute to this work through their own experiences. I would like to thank the authors who shared their intellectual and practical expertise and experiences. I also want to thank the staff at IntechOpen, especially Ms. Marica Novakovic and Ms. Jelena Germuth, for their assistance, competence and patience, without which the publication of this book would not have been possible.

I would like to thank my muse, Barbara, for her support every day.

> *"Culture is the name for what people are interested in, their thoughts, their models, the books they read and the speeches they hear."*
>
> *- Waller Lippmann*

**Andrea Sanna**
Department of General Surgery,
Saint Mary of Angels Hospital,
Adria, Italy

Aulss 5 Polesana,
Rovigo, Italy

Section 1

# Imaging

Chapter 1

# Introductory Chapter: Esophageal Cancer – Current Practice

*Enrico Piva and Andrea Sanna*

## 1. Introduction

Esophageal cancer as a part of upper GI cancers represents the VI leading cause of death for cancer worldwide. The overall 5-year survival rate is from 15 to 25% [1].

Histology of esophageal cancers are various; however, the two major histological subtypes are squamous cell carcinoma (SCC) and adenocarcinoma (AC). Differences in epidemiological distribution of these two major subtypes are observed in eastern and western countries: In east Asia and eastern and southern Africa, SCC has higher prevalence; differently from western countries where prevalence of AC is higher, it is continuously increasing [2, 3].

Esophageal cancer's treatments depend on stage at diagnosis and go from endoscopic resections to conversion surgery for metastatic disease.

Multidisciplinary approach and tailored surgery after multimodal treatment have strongly become current standard for esophageal cancer and R0 intended esophagectomy and continue to play a central role, despite high morbidity and mortality related to these procedures [4].

Effectiveness and oncological adequacy of minimally invasive surgical strategies strengthened their role in multimodal treatment.

## 2. Early stage and endoscopic resection

Endoscopic resection (ER) for esophageal cancer has become a standard for both AC and SCC confined within lamina propria (≤ stage IB) and with low propensity of lymph node metastasis. Nevertheless, in AC data for esophageal cancer lymph node metastasis propensity showed less consistency [5].

A recent study found that for AC lesion >30 mm propensity for submucosal invasion and lymph node invasion was higher and was defined as relative indication for ER, together with the submucosal layer invasion <200 μm. Endoscopic experience, epidemiology of early cancers in east Asia, and precise and accurate studies in eastern countries lead eastern surgeons to expand indications for ER with good oncological outcomes.

Japan Clinical Oncology Group (JCOG) reported a trial 0508 results for ER followed by CRT in patients with SCC staged Ic and they concluded that their strategy was an adequate and effective alternative for R0 esophagectomy in these patients [6].

## 3. Squamous cell carcinoma treatment strategy

Treatment strategies for SCC, because of its lower propensity of hematogenous metastasization and serosa spreading attitude, have developed differently from AC ones, according to evidences.

National Comprehensive Cancer Network (NCCN) Guideline, European Society for Medical Oncology Clinical practice guidelines, and Japanese guidelines consider standard for Esophageal cancer staged cT1-2 N0M0 upfront surgery subordinately for the assessment of adequacy of the patient to elective major surgery. In patients unfit for surgery or not willing to undergo major surgery, definitive CRT should be recommended [7–9].

Treatment for locally advanced resectable SCC has strongly become multimodal and in western country CROSS trial stated a milestone for esophageal cancer treatment. Other scheme for neoadjuvant CT-CRT and adjuvant strategies have been investigated and entered in current practice [9–15].

SCC differently from AC has a specific radiosensitivity and often after neoadjuvant CRT complete pathological response (CPR) has been reported (ypT0N0). The preSANO trial was a prospective multicenter diagnostic cohort study, which aims to establish the accuracy of detection of residual diseases after neoadjuvant CRT. The study showed that endoscopic ultrasonography, bite-on-bite biopsies, and fine needle aspiration (FNA) of lymph nodes were adequate techniques to detect locoregional residue disease together with PET CT for distant metastases. Based on this evidences, a phase III trial (SANO trial) is trying to propose definitive CRT for locally advanced esophageal SCC in patient with complete clinical response (CCR), and this will lead to new approaches for patients unfit for surgery and question the indication for major resection in fit patients as well [16–18].

In patients affected by initially unresectable SCC, conversion surgery has entered in current practice [18].

Resectability of an extended locally advanced disease or oligometastatic disease after neoadjuvant strategy has shown good overall survival (OS) and disease-free survival (DFS) in many different solid tumors' surgery. Although in colorectal surgery conversion therapy is commonly performed, significance of this approach for esophageal cancer is still under debate and lack of strong evidences [19, 20].

## 4. Adenocarcinoma treatment strategy

Adenocarcinoma is the prevalent histology in western countries and experiences differ with eastern ones [21].

Often adenocarcinomas concern to esophagus gastric junction EGJ and localization that slightly differs from thoracic and cervical location because of their different propensity of lymph node metastasization in abdominal district. Siewert classification differentiates type I above Z 2 cm above Z line, type II within 2 cm above Z line and 3 cm below it, and type III below 3 cm of Z line. Studies showed that Siewert III lymph node metastasization was more similar to gastric cancer than what Siewert I and II were [22, 23].

These evidences reflect on current multimodal strategy in which CRT plays a central role as in SCC did, but for distal EGJ AD perioperative CT strategy similar to gastric cancer gave marvelous results [10–12, 24–26].

In surgical strategies, these evidences in lymph node metastasis attitude and tropism for peritoneal spreading reflect in needing for mandatory preoperative laparoscopy for peritoneal assessment and accurate abdominal lymphadenectomy strategy.

## 5. Technique: focus on minimally invasive surgery

Minimally invasive esophagectomy (MIE) has slowly become standard in current practice after evidences about its safety and oncological adequacy.

Two randomized controlled trial were conducted about MIE. The TIME trial compared MIE versus open esophagectomy (OE) in patients affected by cT1-3, N0-1, M0 esophageal cancer evaluating pulmonary complication surgery related, quality of life (QOL), and hospital length of stay (LOS) [27]. Results showed lower ratio for pulmonary complication in MIE arm and better outcomes in terms of LOS and QOL. 3-year follow-up showed no differences in DFS or OS for OS vs. MIE [28].

The other randomized controlled trial was MIRO trial, which investigated transthoracic open procedure versus hybrid minimally invasive procedure (hMIE—laparoscopy and thoracotomy) in patients who underwent subtotal Ivor-Lewis esophagectomy. Complications according to Clavien Dindo grade II or higher were assessed [29]. No differences in survival secondary outcomes and in complications rate between the two groups were assessed.

Currently, a phase III trial compares MIE and OE in ongoing [30].

Another MIE approach described is mediastinoscopy-assisted trans hiatal esophagectomy (MATHE), procedure that avoids single lung ventilation and seems to decrease pulmonary post-operative complications [31].

Robot-assisted surgery is a current practice in surgical oncology worldwide and robot-assisted MIE (RAMIE) has become a standard.

ROBOT trial is the only single-center randomized controlled trial comparing OE and RAMIE with primary endpoint overall complication rate (Clavien Dindo II or Higher). The overall complication rate resulted to be lower in patients underwent RAMIE procedure than OE [32]. RAMIE cost effectiveness is still in debate.

## Author details

Enrico Piva[1,2] and Andrea Sanna[1,2]*

1 Department of General Surgery, Saint Mary of Angels Hospital, Adria, Italy

2 Aulss 5 Polesana, Rovigo, Italy

*Address all correspondence to: and_sanna@yahoo.it

## References

[1] Pennathur A, Gibson MK, Jobe BA, Luketich JD. Oesophageal carcinoma. Lancet. 2013;**381**(9864):400-412. DOI: 10.1016/S0140-6736(12)60643-6

[2] Huang FL, Yu SJ. Esophageal cancer: Risk factors, genetic association, and treatment. Asian Journal of Surgery. 2018;**41**(3):210-215. DOI: 10.1016/j.asjsur.2016.10.005

[3] Watanabe M. Recent topics and perspectives on esophageal cancer in Japan. JMA Journal. 2018;**1**(1):30-39. DOI: 10.31662/jmaj.2018-0002

[4] Takeuchi H, Miyata H, Gotoh M, et al. A risk model for esophagectomy using data of 5354 patients included in a Japanese nationwide web-based database. Annals of Surgery. 2014;**260**(2):259-266. DOI: 10.1097/SLA.0000000000000644

[5] Ishihara R, Oyama T, Abe S, et al. Risk of metastasis in adenocarcinoma of the esophagus: A multicenter retrospective study in a Japanese population. Journal of Gastroenterology. 2017;**52**(7):800-808. DOI: 10.1007/s00535-016-1275-0

[6] Minashi K, Nihei K, Mizusawa J, et al. Efficacy of endoscopic resection and selective chemoradiotherapy for stage I esophageal squamous cell carcinoma. Gastroenterology. 2019;**157**(2):382-390.e3. DOI: 10.1053/j.gastro.2019.04.017

[7] Ajani JA, D'Amico TA, Bentrem DJ, et al. Esophageal and esophagogastric junction cancers, version 2.2019. JNCCN Journal of the National Comprehensive Cancer Network. 2019;**17**(7):855-883. DOI: 10.6004/jnccn.2019.0033

[8] Lordick F, Mariette C, Haustermans K, Obermannová R, Arnold D, on behalf of the ESMO Guidelines Committee clinicalguidelines@esmo org. Oesophageal cancer: ESMO clinical practice guidelines for diagnosis, treatment and follow-up. Annals of Oncology. 2016;**27**(2003):v50-v57. DOI: 10.1093/annonc/mdw329

[9] Kitagawa Y, Uno T, Oyama T, et al. Esophageal cancer practice guidelines 2017 edited by the Japan esophageal society: Part 1. Esophagus. 2019;**16**(1): 1-24. DOI: 10.1007/s10388-018-0641-9

[10] van Hagen P, Hulshof MCCM, van Lanschot JJB, et al. Preoperative Chemoradiotherapy for esophageal or junctional cancer. The New England Journal of Medicine. 2012;**366**(22):2074-2084. DOI: 10.1056/nejmoa1112088

[11] Shapiro J, van Lanschot JJB, Hulshof MCCM, et al. Neoadjuvant chemoradiotherapy plus surgery versus surgery alone for oesophageal or junctional cancer (CROSS): Long-term results of a randomised controlled trial. The Lancet Oncology. 2015;**16**(9):1090-1098. DOI: 10.1016/S1470-2045(15)00040-6

[12] Pasini F, de Manzoni G, Pedrazzani C, et al. High pathological response rate in locally advanced esophageal cancer after neoadjuvant combined modality therapy: Dose finding of a weekly chemotherapy schedule with protracted venous infusion of 5-fluorouracil and dose escalation of cisplatin, docetaxel and concurrent radiotherapy. Annals of Oncology. 2005;**16**(7):1133-1139. DOI: 10.1093/annonc/mdi207

[13] Ando N, Kato H, Igaki H, et al. A randomized trial comparing postoperative adjuvant chemotherapy

with cisplatin and 5-fluorouracil versus preoperative chemotherapy for localized advanced squamous cell carcinoma of the thoracic esophagus (JCOG9907). Annals of Surgical Oncology. 2012;**19**(1):68-74. DOI: 10.1245/s10434-011-2049-9

[14] Ando N, Iizuka T, Ide H, et al. Surgery plus chemotherapy compared with surgery alone for localized squamous cell carcinoma of the thoracic esophagus: A Japan clinical oncology group study - JCOG9204. Journal of Clinical Oncology. 2003;**21**(24):4592-4596. DOI: 10.1200/JCO.2003.12.095

[15] Nakamura K, Kato K, Igaki H, et al. Three-arm phase III trial comparing cisplatin plus 5-FU (CF) versus docetaxel, cisplatin plus 5-FU (DCF) versus radiotherapy with CF (CF-RT) as preoperative therapy for locally advanced esophageal cancer (JCOG1109, NExT study). Japanese Journal of Clinical Oncology. 2013;**43**(7):752-755. DOI: 10.1093/jjco/hyt061

[16] Noordman BJ, Spaander MCW, Valkema R, et al. Detection of residual disease after neoadjuvant chemoradiotherapy for oesophageal cancer (preSANO): A prospective multicentre, diagnostic cohort study. The Lancet Oncology. 2018;**19**(7):965-974. DOI: 10.1016/S1470-2045(18)30201-8

[17] Noordman BJ, Wijnhoven BPL, Lagarde SM, et al. Neoadjuvant chemoradiotherapy plus surgery versus active surveillance for oesophageal cancer: A stepped-wedge cluster randomised trial. BMC Cancer. 2018;**18**(1):1-12. DOI: 10.1186/s12885-018-4034-1

[18] Yoshida K, Yamaguchi K, Okumura N, Tanahashi T, Kodera Y. Is conversion therapy possible in stage IV gastric cancer: The proposal of new biological categories of classification. Gastric Cancer. 2016;**19**(2):329-338. DOI: 10.1007/s10120-015-0575-z

[19] Yokota T, Kato K, Hamamoto Y, et al. Phase II study of chemoselection with docetaxel plus cisplatin and 5-fluorouracil induction chemotherapy and subsequent conversion surgery for locally advanced unresectable oesophageal cancer. British Journal of Cancer. 2016;**115**(11):1328-1334. DOI: 10.1038/bjc.2016.350

[20] Terada M, Hara H, Daiko H, et al. Phase III study of tri-modality combination therapy with induction docetaxel plus cisplatin and 5-fluorouracil versus definitive chemoradiotherapy for locally advanced unresectable squamous-cell carcinoma of the thoracic esophagus (JCOG1510: TRIANgLE). Japanese Journal of Clinical Oncology. 2019;**49**(11):1055-1060. DOI: 10.1093/jjco/hyz112

[21] Giacopuzzi S, Bencivenga M, Weindelmayer J, Verlato G, de Manzoni G. Western strategy for EGJ carcinoma. Gastric Cancer. 2017;**20**:60-68. DOI: 10.1007/s10120-016-0685-2

[22] Pedrazzani C, de Manzoni G, Marrelli D, et al. Lymph node involvement in advanced gastroesophageal junction adenocarcinoma. The Journal of Thoracic and Cardiovascular Surgery. 2007;**134**(2):378-385. DOI: 10.1016/j.jtcvs.2007.03.034

[23] Mine S, Kurokawa Y, Takeuchi H, et al. Distribution of involved abdominal lymph nodes is correlated with the distance from the esophagogastric junction to the distal end of the tumor in Siewert type II tumors. European Journal of Surgical Oncology. 2015;**41**(10):1348-1353. DOI: 10.1016/j.ejso.2015.05.004

[24] Zanoni A, Verlato G, Giacopuzzi S, et al. Neoadjuvant

concurrent chemoradiotherapy for locally advanced esophageal cancer in a single high-volume center. Annals of Surgical Oncology. 2013;**20**(6):1993-1999. DOI: 10.1245/s10434-012-2822-4

[25] Allum WH, Stenning SP, Bancewicz J, Clark PI, Langley RE. Long-term results of a randomized trial of surgery with or without preoperative chemotherapy in esophageal cancer. Journal of Clinical Oncology. 2009;**27**(30):5062-5067. DOI: 10.1200/JCO.2009.22.2083

[26] Al-Batran SE, Homann N, Pauligk C, et al. Perioperative chemotherapy with fluorouracil plus leucovorin, oxaliplatin, and docetaxel versus fluorouracil or capecitabine plus cisplatin and epirubicin for locally advanced, resectable gastric or gastro-oesophageal junction adenocarcinoma (FLOT4): A randomised, phase 2/3 trial. Lancet. 2019;**393**(10184):1948-1957. DOI: 10.1016/S0140-6736(18)32557-1

[27] Biere SSAY, Van Berge Henegouwen MI, Maas KW, et al. Minimally invasive versus open oesophagectomy for patients with oesophageal cancer: A multicentre, open-label, randomised controlled trial. Lancet. 2012;**379**(9829):1887-1892. DOI: 10.1016/S0140-6736(12)60516-9

[28] Straatman J, Van Der Wielen N, Cuesta MA, et al. Minimally invasive versus open esophageal resection. Annals of Surgery. 2017;**266**(2):232-236. DOI: 10.1097/SLA.0000000000002171

[29] Mariette C, Markar SR, Dabakuyo-Yonli TS, et al. Hybrid minimally invasive Esophagectomy for esophageal cancer. The New England Journal of Medicine. 2019;**380**(2):152-162. DOI: 10.1056/nejmoa1805101

[30] Kataoka K, Takeuchi H, Mizusawa J, et al. A randomized phase III trial of thoracoscopic versus open esophagectomy for thoracic esophageal cancer: Japan clinical oncology group study JCOG1409. Japanese Journal of Clinical Oncology. 2016;**46**(2):174-177. DOI: 10.1093/jjco/hyv178

[31] Feng MX, Wang H, Zhang Y, Tan LJ, Xu ZL, Qun W. Minimally invasive esophagectomy for esophageal squamous cell carcinoma: A case-control study of thoracoscope versus mediastinoscope assistance. Surgical Endoscopy. 2012;**26**(6):1573-1578. DOI: 10.1007/s00464-011-2073-7

[32] van der Sluis PC, van der Horst S, May AM, et al. Robot-assisted minimally invasive Thoracolaparoscopic Esophagectomy versus open transthoracic Esophagectomy for Resectable esophageal cancer: A randomized controlled trial. Annals of Surgery. 2019;**269**(4):621-630. DOI: 10.1097/SLA.0000000000003031

Chapter 2

# Scope of Real Time Fluorescence Imaging in Esophagectomy

*Subramanyeshwar Rao Thammineedi, Srijan Shukla, Nusrath Syed, Ajesh Raj Saksena, Sujit Chyau Patnaik and Pratap Reddy Ramalingam*

## Abstract

Esophagectomy is a challenging surgery that is known to be associated with high rates of morbidity. Anastomotic leaks, pneumonia, conduit necrosis and chyle leaks are the commonly reported complications. Perfusion assessment and tissue injection based fluorescence guided surgery (FGS) are the newer clinical applications of fluorescent dyes. With the advent and integration of real time fluorescence imaging with the existing minimal access platforms, the esophageal surgeon can employ these techniques to potentially improve outcomes. During thoracic dissection, thoracic duct lymphography, fluorescence guided airway visualization, tracheal perfusion assessment and sentinel lymph node biopsy/dissection are the reported clinical applications. In the abdominal dissection, gastroepiploic arcade identification, gastric conduit perfusion assessment and proximal esophagus perfusion assessment have been described. Using the different routes of administration, the same dye can be used for different uses at separate points in a single esophagectomy surgery. The principles and evidence pertaining to these applications have been outlined.

**Keywords:** esophagectomy, indocyanine green, ICG, fluorescence imaging, near infrared, thoracic duct, gastric conduit

## 1. Introduction

Real time fluorescence imaging with indocyanine green (ICG) is a promising technology with a potential to resolve many challenges during esophagectomy including the assessment of gastric conduit vascularity, ICG-guided navigation surgery for an adequate lymphadenectomy, detection of sentinel nodes in early stage cancer, defining trachea and bronchial tree and in delineating thoracic duct anatomy and identification of chyle leaks during and after surgery [1]. It is also useful in identifying and safeguarding gastroepiploic arcade vital for gastric conduit creation, especially in obese patients where arcade detection could be challenging. This article provides an overview of the principles of fluorescence imaging, types of fluorescence dyes, indications of fluorescence-guided surgery (FGS) and summarizes the utility of FGS in relation to esophageal surgery.

## 2. Near-infrared fluorescence- the physics

Intraoperative fluorescence utilizes the property of specific molecules which absorb light at a particular wavelength and emit light at a longer wavelength [2]. When stimulated by an external light source, these molecules are excited, and the emission occurs at a longer wavelength in the near-infrared range (NIR) (650–900 nm). The emitted light is captured using a camera equipped with specialized filters, and the visualization of the fluorescence signal is relayed to an external display providing real-time in vivo imaging.

The light emitted in the NIR spectrum cannot be seen by human eyes. The NIR fluorescent cameras selectively capture it. Also, NIR fluorescence has the advantages of low background autofluorescence from blood components (hemoglobin and water) and an excellent signal-to-background ratio, providing clear fluorescence visuals.

## 3. Fluorescent dyes- the chemistry

Fluorescein, 5-amino levulinic acid, indocyanine green (ICG), and methylene blue are fluorescent dyes used for in vivo fluorescent imaging. Indocyanine green, small diameter water soluble tricarbocyanine dye, exhibits fluorescence when activated by NIR light within the wavelength of 760 to 780 nm delivered by a near-infrared optical system. On excitation, ICG emits a fluorescence emission between 800 and 850 nm, which the NIR device captures [3]. The depth of tissue visualization varies between 0.5 and 1 cm. When injected intravenously, ICG is tightly bound to the plasma proteins and remains within the intravascular compartment. This property is helpful for angiography assessment of the gastric conduit or tissue perfusion. It rapidly washes out with a short half-life of 150–180 seconds. When injected submucosal or intranodal, ICG is distributed through the lymphatic system. ICG concentrates in the liver and is excreted through the biliary system, which helps delineate the biliary system for fluorescence cholangiography. ICG is relatively safe with a low risk of adverse effects at a dose of 0.1 mg to 0.5 mg/mL/kg for human use [4]. Methylene blue (MB) is a thiazine dye and has also shown to have fluorescent properties. It has an excitation peak of approximately 700 nm with less tissue penetration but more background tissue autofluorescence. It can be administered orally, subcutaneously, or intravenously. MB is excreted through the kidneys and is contraindicated in patients with renal insufficiency [5].

## 4. Routes of administration- the biology

The versatility of fluorescent dyes has opened up many interesting clinical applications. The route of administration of the dye determines the drainage pathway of the dye. The resultant highlighted structures can help the surgeon make the intended surgical decisions (**Table 1**). The most commonly used route is the intravenous injection wherein the perfusion of the organ under interest has to be studied. ICG has been successfully studied in assessment of perfusion of anastomotic segments of colon, rectum and esophagus [6]. Because the predominant excretion of ICG happens via the biliary tract, delayed fluorescence imaging performed upto 15 hours after injection allows for cholangiography [7]. When ICG is injected directly into tissues, it gets drained by nearby lymphatic channels to the regional lymph node. This concept

| Route of administration | Intended use | Clinical application |
|---|---|---|
| Intravenous | Perfusion assessment | Gastric conduit perfusion (esophagectomy), Flap perfusion (reconstructive surgery, Colon perfusion (Colectomy) |
| Intravenous | Biliary drainage | Cholangiography |
| Peritumoral | Lymph node mapping | Sentinel lymph node biopsy (Breast carcinoma, endometrial carcinoma) |
| Groin nodal injection | Lymphography | Chyle leak localization, Thoracic duct mapping |
| Aerosol inhalation/ nebulisation | Airway fluorescence | To be studied |

**Table 1.**
*Various routes of administration of fluorescence dyes and their clinical applications.*

is utilized in sentinel lymph node biopsy (SLNB). Peritumoral ICG injection has been found to be a suitable alternative to other dyes in breast and endometrial carcinoma [8, 9]. Lymphatic system of retroperitoneum and thoracic duct can be imaged via ICG injection in groin lymph node. This has opened up a new avenue to visualize and manage thoracic duct and chyle leaks [10, 11]. Fluorescein aerosolization has been attempted and fluorescence confirmed on thoracoscopy [12]. Further studies are required to explore the administration of fluorescent dyes via airway.

## 5. Technology integration

Recent advances in esophagectomy include wide acceptance of minimal access surgery (MAS) approaches. MAS reduced the major morbidity associated with esophagectomy with equivalent oncological outcomes. With MAS came the advantages of magnification and better identification of surgical anatomy. To improve upon the previous iterations of camera systems, newer cameras have integrated fluorescence imaging capabilities. The first generation fluorescence integrated cameras required the surgeon to switch off white light and the fluorescent structure would get highlighted in a background of darkness. Second generation fluorescence integrated cameras overcame this by adding artificial intelligence to overlay the fluorescent structure over a well-lit background. This enabled interruption free instrumentation and accurate dissection. Portable handheld cameras with integrated fluorescence capabilities are also available now for open surgeries. With these modern adjuncts in the armamentarium, an esophageal surgeon stands at an advantage of having real time information pertaining to various critical steps of an otherwise complex procedure.

The technology has been increasingly utilized for real-time surgical decision-making. Various commercially available equipment for open, laparoscopic, and robotic platforms simultaneously provides high-definition fluorescence and white light images on the same screen. These systems have built-in NIR filters, a camera, and a visual processor for capturing high-definition fluorescent images. The fluorescence and white light modes can be conveniently toggled by clicking a button or using a foot pedal switch (**Table 2**) [5].

| Open procedures | Thoracoscopy/Laparoscopy | Robotic platforms |
|---|---|---|
| • PDE- Neo II<br>• Quest Spectrum<br>• Stryker PINPOINT with SPY-PHI | • Karl Storz IMAGE 1 S™/ IMAGE 1 S™ Rubina<br>• Quest Spectrum<br>• Stryker 1688 AIM | • Da Vinci Surgical Systems with Firefly |

**Table 2.**
*Commercially available integrated fluorescence imaging platforms.*

## 6. Challenges in esophagectomy

Esophagectomy is a complex surgery requiring the surgeon to master both technical and cognitive skills. MAS approaches have their own learning curves and learning curve associated complications have also been reported [13, 14]. The major challenges for a team managing esophagectomy patients include prevention and management of these postoperative complications. Pneumonia, anastomotic leaks, chylothorax, conduit necrosis are the most often reported complications [15]. Patients who experience major complications tend to have poorer overall survival as well [15]. Predictive factors for anastomotic leaks have been studied and apart from the medical comorbidities of the patient, technique of surgery has also been found to be a significant risk factor [16]. It is generally accepted that ensuring and improving adequate blood supply affects leak rates in esophageal anastomoses [17]. Visual assessment of gastric conduit perfusion is considered inadequate [18]. Fluorescence perfusion assessment offers opportunity to study real time blood supply to the anastomotic segments.

During thoracic dissection in esophagectomy, thoracic duct is a difficult structure to appreciate under white light. As radiation therapy before surgery is being increasingly used for locally advanced tumors, the tissue planes can get fused making identification of thoracic duct even harder. Chylothorax can be very debilitating and may increase length of stay and mortality rates [19]. Fluorescence lymphography is being explored for accurate intraoperative identification of thoracic duct [11, 20]. Newer morphological patterns of thoracic duct previously not described are also being reported [20].

## 7. Thoracic duct lymphangiography

Chylothorax after thoracic surgeries is an infrequent postoperative complication. Incidence of chylothorax ranges from 1.4% after transthoracic esophageal resection to 2.4% after transhiatal esophagectomy [21]. Thoracic duct injury is a serious complication after chest surgery and major neck dissections that significantly increases hospital stay, with high in-hospital mortality [22–25]. Chyle leak carries high morbidity up to 38% and mortality as high as 25% [26].

The non-visualization of the thoracic duct with its proximity to the esophagus makes it prone to iatrogenic injury during surgery, leading to chylothorax. The diagnosis is considered in the presence of excessive pleural output and established by biochemical and physical characteristics of the fluid. Intraoperative identification of the thoracic duct can be difficult, especially during reoperation. Because traditional conservative treatment of thoracic duct injury has a high failure rate, intraoperative image guidance is essential for proper surgical management. Presently, lymphoscintigraphy and lymphangiography are available in preoperative setting to diagnose and recognize the site of thoracic duct injury; however, these procedures cannot accurately guide the surgeon during surgery [27, 28]. Oral administration of heavy cream before surgery is sometimes performed to visualize chyle leak [29].

Real time fluorescence imaging with ICG has the potential to solve all these issues. Thoracic duct NIR fluorescence imaging with ICG has been reported earlier for the recognition of site of chyle leak after esophageal and other thoracic surgeries in form of case reports [11, 30]. Using subcutaneous ICG injection at the inguinal area, Chang et al. identified and ligated chyle leak site through re-sternotomy in a 3-month-old infant with congenital heart disease who had refractory postoperative chylothorax despite multiple line of managements [31]. Kaburagi et al. performed successful mass ligation of thoracic duct at the level of the diaphragmatic crura following ICG injection in mesentery in a case of post esophagectomy chyle leak [32].

Vecchiato et al. reported their experience of minimally invasive esophagectomy with ICG injection in inguinal lymph nodes in 19 patients. The thoracic duct was identified in all patients after a mean of 52.7 minutes from injection time [11]. The protocol followed at the author's surgical unit is as follows. After induction of anesthesia, ICG is injected in groin node with ultrasound guidance. ICG is available as 25 mg powder (Aurogreen; Aurolabs, Madurai, India), which is reconstituted in 10 ml of sterile distilled water. One ml of the solution contains 2.5 mg of ICG. One ml is injected via ultrasound guidance in a groin node, one each on both sides. Generally, the node appears as an oval structure in ultrasound with central echoic and peripheral hypoechoic architecture. A successful administration is noted by tumescence of the node with loss of central hyperechoic architecture. Real time fluorescence lymphography is utilized at the time of thoracic dissection (**Figure 1**). Thoracic duct is visualized and safeguarded in all cases of esophagectomy, unless directly involved by the tumor (**Figure 2**) [1].

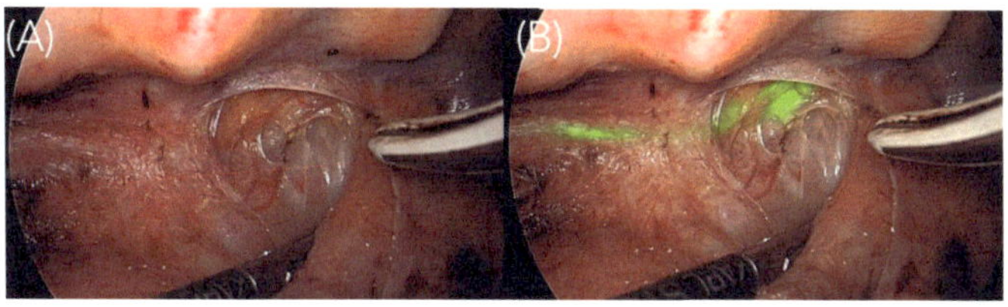


**Figure 1.**
*Comparison of thoracic duct visualization without and with real time fluorescence lymphography. (A) White light thoracoscopy with esophagus retracted towards surgeon to stretch mesoesophagus to allow for visualization of thoracic duct. (B) Real time fluorescence lymphography turned on, thoracic duct along its course is highlighted.*

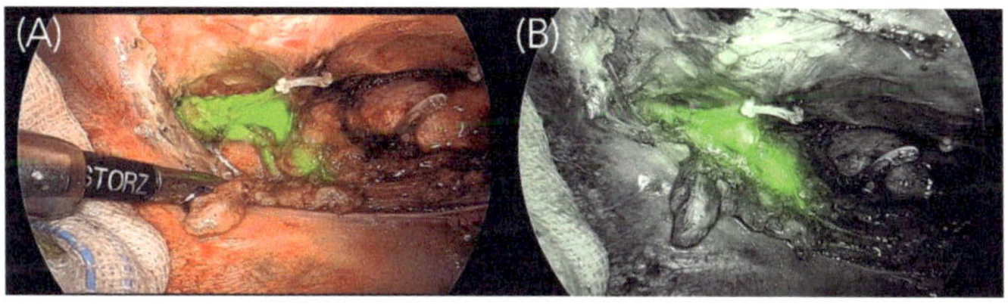


**Figure 2.**
*Real time fluorescence lymphography depicting thoracic duct involvement by lower third esophageal carcinoma under different modes. (A) Overlay mode. (B) Color segmented fluorescence (CSF) mode.*

## 8. Fluorescence nebulization for airway visualization

In locally advanced upper and mid thoracic esophageal cancers, the posterior plane of dissection is limited by the membranous trachea. Bulky subcarinal and hilar lymph nodes can also pose difficulty in dissection over posterior surface of right and left bronchi. The fear of injuring the tracheobronchial membrane makes this part of thoracic dissection in esophagectomy an extremely challenging task. Fluorescence guided airway visualization could be an adjunct in this regard.

Thoracic surgeons have utilized ICG for determining the intersegmental plane in lung segmentectomies [33]. While intravenous ICG injection was studied initially, subsequently endobronchial injection has also been successfully attempted [34]. The authors have applied the same principle by performing nebulization of ICG for early visualization and accurate dissection of posterior membrane of trachea and bronchus in difficult tumors. Using the overlay mode of the NIR camera, esophagus and the lymph nodes can be safely separated from the highlighted membranous trachea and bronchus. **Figure 3** illustrates this technique. Fluorescence nebulization is being tested as a prospective study to standardize the application and evaluate the safety and potential advantages.

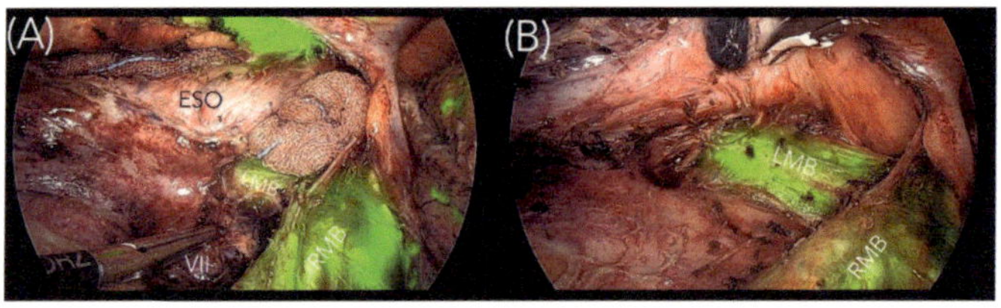


**Figure 3.**
*Fluorescence nebulization and airway visualization. (A) Middle third esophageal tumor (ESO) with contiguous bulky subcarinal lymph node (VII). Right main bronchus (RMB) is dissected away. Left main bronchus (LMB) remains to be dissected, posterior surface is starting to come into view and is highlighted via fluorescence. (B) Subcarinal lymphadenectomy and ventral dissection of esophagus over LMB is complete.*

## 9. Sentinel nodal mapping and guided lymphadenectomy

Real time fluorescence imaging can be used for lymphatic mapping in esophageal cancer to better delineate the lymphatic pathways and to aid nodal dissection. Yuasa et al. determined the feasibility of sentinel lymph node (SLN) detection using intraoperative ICG fluorescence imaging navigated by preoperative computed tomographic lymphography (CTLG) in 20 superficial esophageal cancer patients. Preoperative CTLG localized the number and site of SLNs during computed tomography. Further, SLNs were identified intraoperatively, resulting in successful SLN navigation [35]. Schlottmann et al. and Hachey et al. demonstrated the feasibility of sentinel nodal mapping in patients with esophagogastric junction and mid third esophageal malignancies [36, 37]. Schlottmann et al. identified the pattern of nodal drainage by submucosal injection of 2.5 mg ICG via endoscopy in 4 peritumoral quadrants 15–20 minutes before surgery. Left gastric nodes were the first lymph node station to exhibit fluorescence in 8 out of 9 cases. Hachey et al. utilized ICG: human serum albumin (ICG: HSA) to better delineate nodes with near infrared indocyanine green (NIR-ICG). In order to improve fluorescence-guided sentinel lymph node biopsy, Kim et al., in an animal model, used a novel macrophage-targeting ICG bound to human serum albumin (ICG:MSA). This ICG:MSA compound when injected via endoscopy into esophageal tissue has provided promising results in sentinel lymph node detection in a porcine model [38].

## 10. Gastric conduit perfusion assessment

One of the most feared complications post esophagectomy is anastomotic leak (AL), occurring in 10–30% of patients [39]. While fashioning the gastric conduit, both left gastric and short gastric vessels are usually divided. The conduit solely relies on the right gastroepiploic artery for its blood supply. Inadequate perfusion at the tip of the gastric conduit is one of the most critical factors contributing to anastomotic leak. Conventional assessment techniques of the perfusion and viability of gastric conduit such as visual inspection of the gastric conduit color, warmth, pulsation of the arcade and bleed from the cut edges are considered unreliable. Accurate assessment of perfusion and selecting an appropriate anastomotic site are critical to reduce AL [40]. As a means of evaluating blood flow, indocyanine green (ICG) fluorescence angiography (FA) has recently been introduced to provide real-time assessment of the anastomotic area during esophagectomy [18]. ICG can be used as a vascular contrast agent for assessing perfusion of gastric conduit (**Figure 4**) [5].

A meta-analysis by Slooter et al. reported that ICG significantly decreases anastomotic leaks and graft necrosis after esophagectomy (OR 0.30, 95% CI: 0.14–0.63). The pooled change in management rate due to fluorescence angiography using ICG was 24.55%. Change in management included excision of the poorly perfused area of the gastric conduit and change in site of anastomosis. Despite the change in management, the pooled incidence of anastomotic leak and graft necrosis was as high as 14.08% [41]. Another meta-analysis by Degett et al. reported similar anastomotic leak rate (14%) in patients with esophageal anastomoses after intraoperative ICG fluorescence angiographic assessment [42].

Time to fluorescence is an important parameter which has been studied. The data pertaining to this aspect of the fluorescence angiography is heterogenous.

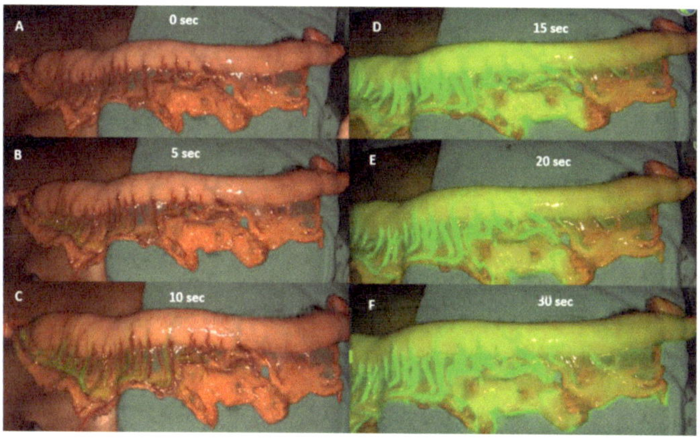


**Figure 4.**
*Real time fluorescence perfusion assessment of gastric conduit. (A-F) fluorescence perfusion assessed at various time intervals after intravenous injection of indocyanine green (ICG) dye.*

Ishige et al. studied different patterns of time to fluorescence intensity curves. They found a "normal" pattern, characterized by a sharp high peak in fluorescence intensity in gastric tubes followed by rapid decline to plateau level, prior to division of perigastric vessels in 6 cases (30%). The other 14 cases showed a "gradual" pattern, characterized by an obtuse and low arterial inflow peak and slow increase in fluorescence intensity over time. However, no anastomotic leak occurred in both groups [43]. Yukaya et al. described three types of curves, normal, outflow delayed and an inflow delayed. Anastomotic leak occurred in 23.1% (3/13) in the normal type, 40% (2/5) in the outflow delayed type and 44.4% (4/9) in the inflow delayed type, with no significant difference among the three types [44]. Koyanagi et al. stratified patients into two groups according to ICG fluorescence flow speed: a simultaneous group with identical speed in gastric conduit wall and the greater curvature vessels, and a delayed group where the ICG fluorescence was slower in the gastric conduit wall in comparison to the greater curvature vessels. They calculated a threshold ICG flow speed of 1.76 cm/s in the gastric conduit predicting anastomotic leak. None of the patients developed anastomotic leak in the simultaneous group, while it occurred in 47% (7/15) patients in the delayed group [45]. Kumagai et al. proposed a 90-second rule wherein all anastomoses were to be reconstructed in the area that showed an enhancement within 90 seconds after initial enhancement at the root of the right gastroepiploic artery [19]. The tip needed revision in 50% (35/70), and in 18 of those 35 patients, a change in anastomotic site was needed. Anastomotic leak occured in 1 out of 70 cases (1.4%) [46]. Slooter et al. reported that the time between ICG injection and enhancement of tip was not significantly prolonged in patients with an anastomotic leak versus no leak (63 vs. 45 seconds) ($P = 0.066$) and time to fluorescence from base of conduit to the planned anastomosis was significantly increased in patients with a postoperative anastomotic stricture (13 vs. 7 seconds [47].

Nakashima et al. described outcomes of fluorescence angiography assessment of the pedicled omental flap performed to reinforce the esophagogastric anastomosis. Poorly perfused omental tissue was excised on the demarcation line. Anastomotic leak and stricture occurred in 1/38 (2.6%) and 2/38 (5.3%) patients respectively [48]. The importance of proximal esophageal stump revision has been emphasized by Thammineedi et al. where 5 out of 13 patients (38.46%) underwent revision of proximal esophageal stump after ICG assessment [18]. Randomized controlled trials are warranted to prove the exact benefit of ICG fluorescence angiography in reducing anastomotic leaks and strictures in esophagectomy.

## 11. Future directions

Fluorescent dyes have been around for more than 40 years [3]. In the past decade interest has grown especially after incorporation of fluorescence capable MAS platforms. Most studies of fluorescence guided surgery have been single center experiences. Multicenter trials with better study designs are needed. International collaborations between societies can lead to standardization of techniques and uniform reporting of outcomes.

## Conflict of interest

The authors declare no conflict of interest.

## Author details

Subramanyeshwar Rao Thammineedi, Srijan Shukla*, Nusrath Syed,
Ajesh Raj Saksena, Sujit Chyau Patnaik and Pratap Reddy Ramalingam
Department of Surgical Oncology, Basavatarakam Indo American Cancer Hospital and Research Institute, Hyderabad, India

*Address all correspondence to: shuklasrajan@gmail.com

## References


[1] Thammineedi SR, Patnaik SC, Reddy P, Saksena AR, Bollineni N, Nusrath S. The emerging role of ICG fluorescence during minimally invasive Esophagectomy. Indian Journal of Surgical Oncology. 2021;**12**(3):635-636

[2] Weissleder R, Pittet MJ. Imaging in the era of molecular oncology. Nature. 2008;**452**(7187):580-589

[3] Benson RC, Kues HA. Fluorescence properties of indocyanine green as related to angiography. Physics in Medicine and Biology. 1978;**23**(1):159-163

[4] Alander JT, Kaartinen I, Laakso A, Pätilä T, Spillmann T, Tuchin VV, et al. A review of indocyanine green fluorescent imaging in surgery. International Journal of Biomedical Imaging. 2012;**2012**:940585

[5] Thammineedi SR, Saksena AR, Nusrath S, Iyer RR, Shukla S, Patnaik SC, et al. Fluorescence-guided cancer surgery—A new paradigm. Journal of Surgical Oncology. 2021;**123**(8):1679-1698

[6] Blanco-Colino R, Espin-Basany E. Intraoperative use of ICG fluorescence imaging to reduce the risk of anastomotic leakage in colorectal surgery: A systematic review and meta-analysis. Techniques in Coloproctology. 2018;**22**(1):15-23

[7] Tsutsui N, Yoshida M, Nakagawa H, Ito E, Iwase R, Suzuki N, et al. Optimal timing of preoperative indocyanine green administration for fluorescent cholangiography during laparoscopic cholecystectomy using the PINPOINT® endoscopic fluorescence imaging system. Asian Journal of Endoscopic Surgery. 2018;**11**(3):199-205

[8] Grischke EM, Röhm C, Hahn M, Helms G, Brucker S, Wallwiener D. ICG fluorescence technique for the detection of sentinel lymph nodes in breast cancer: Results of a prospective open-label clinical trial. Geburtshilfe und Frauenheilkunde. 2015;**75**(9):935-940

[9] Rossi EC, Kowalski LD, Scalici J, Cantrell L, Schuler K, Hanna RK, et al. A comparison of sentinel lymph node biopsy to lymphadenectomy for endometrial cancer staging (FIRES trial): A multicentre, prospective, cohort study. The Lancet Oncology. 2017;**18**(3):384-392

[10] Shimajiri H, Egi H, Yamamoto M, Kochi M, Mukai S, Ohdan H. Laparoscopic management of refractory chylous ascites using fluorescence navigation with indocyanine green: A case report. International Journal of Surgery Case Reports. 2018;**49**:149-152

[11] Vecchiato M, Martino A, Sponza M, Uzzau A, Ziccarelli A, Marchesi F, et al. Thoracic duct identification with indocyanine green fluorescence during minimally invasive esophagectomy with patient in prone position. Diseases of the Esophagus. 2020;**33**(12):doaa030

[12] Noppen M, Dekeukeleire T, Hanon S, Stratakos G, Amjadi K, Madsen P, et al. Fluorescein-enhanced autofluorescence thoracoscopy in patients with primary spontaneous pneumothorax and normal subjects. American Journal of Respiratory and Critical Care Medicine. 2006;**174**(1):26-30

[13] Prasad P, Wallace L, Navidi M, Phillips AW. Learning curves in minimally invasive esophagectomy: A systematic review and evaluation of

benchmarking parameters. Surgery. 2022;**171**(5):1247-1256

[14] van Workum F, Stenstra MHBC, Berkelmans GHK, Slaman AE, van Berge Henegouwen MI, Gisbertz SS, et al. Learning curve and associated morbidity of minimally invasive Esophagectomy: A retrospective multicenter study. Annals of Surgery. 2019;**269**(1):88-94

[15] Booka E, Takeuchi H, Nishi T, Matsuda S, Kaburagi T, Fukuda K, et al. The impact of postoperative complications on survivals after Esophagectomy for esophageal cancer. Medicine (Baltimore). 2015;**94**(33):e1369

[16] Kassis ES, Kosinski AS, Ross P, Koppes KE, Donahue JM, Daniel VC. Predictors of anastomotic leak after esophagectomy: An analysis of the society of thoracic surgeons general thoracic database. The Annals of Thoracic Surgery. 2013;**96**(6):1919-1926

[17] Reavis KM. The esophageal anastomosis: How improving blood supply affects leak rate. Journal of Gastrointestinal Surgery. 2009;**13**(9):1558-1560

[18] Thammineedi SR, Patnaik SC, Saksena AR, Ramalingam PR, Nusrath S. The utility of Indocyanine green angiography in the assessment of perfusion of gastric conduit and proximal esophageal stump against visual assessment in patients undergoing Esophagectomy: A prospective study. Indian Journal of Surgical Oncology. 2020;**11**(4):684-691

[19] Miao L, Zhang Y, Hu H, Ma L, Shun Y, Xiang J, et al. Incidence and management of chylothorax after esophagectomy. Thoracic Cancer. 2015;**6**(3):354-358

[20] Tokumaru S, Kitazawa M, Nakamura S, Koyama M, Soejima Y. Intraoperative visualization of morphological patterns of the thoracic duct by subcutaneous inguinal injection of indocyanine green in esophagectomy for esophageal cancer. Annals of Gastroenterological Surgery. 2022;**00**:1-7. DOI: 10.1002/ags3.12594

[21] Hulscher JB, Tijssen JG, Obertop H, van Lanschot JJ. Transthoracic versus transhiatal resection for carcinoma of the esophagus: A meta-analysis. The Annals of Thoracic Surgery. 2001;**72**(1):306-313

[22] Brinkmann S, Schroeder W, Junggeburth K, Gutschow CA, Bludau M, Hoelscher AH, et al. Incidence and management of chylothorax after Ivor Lewis esophagectomy for cancer of the esophagus. The Journal of Thoracic and Cardiovascular Surgery. 2016;**151**(5):1398-1404

[23] Lapp GC, Brown DH, Gullane PJ, McKneally M. Thoracoscopic management of chylous fistulae. American Journal of Otolaryngology. 1998;**19**(4):257-262

[24] Wurnig PN, Hollaus PH, Ohtsuka T, Flege JB, Wolf RK. Thoracoscopic direct clipping of the thoracic duct for chylopericardium and chylothorax. The Annals of Thoracic Surgery. 2000;**70**(5):1662-1665

[25] Fahimi H, Casselman FP, Mariani MA, van Boven WJ, Knaepen PJ, van Swieten HA. Current management of postoperative chylothorax. The Annals of Thoracic Surgery. 2001;**71**(2):448-450 discussion 450-451

[26] Schild HH, Strassburg CP, Welz A, Kalff J. Treatment options in patients with chylothorax. Deutsches Ärzteblatt International. 2013;**110**(48):819-826

[27] Kotani K, Kawabe J, Higashiyama S, Shiomi S. Lymphoscintigraphy with

single-photon emission computed tomography/computed tomography is useful for determining the site of chyle leakage after esophagectomy. Indian Journal of Nuclear Medicine: IJNM: The Official Journal of the Society of Nuclear Medicine. 2012;**27**(3):208-209

[28] Sachs PB, Zelch MG, Rice TW, Geisinger MA, Risius B, Lammert GK. Diagnosis and localization of laceration of the thoracic duct: Usefulness of lymphangiography and CT. AJR. American Journal of Roentgenology. 1991;**157**(4):703-705

[29] Shen Y, Feng M, Khan MA, Wang H, Tan L, Wang Q. A simple method minimizes chylothorax after minimally invasive esophagectomy. Journal of the American College of Surgeons. 2014;**218**(1):108-112

[30] Bibas BJ, Costa-de-Carvalho RL, Pola-dos-Reis F, Lauricella LL, Pêgo-Fernandes PM, Terra RM. Video-assisted thoracoscopic thoracic duct ligation with near-infrared fluorescence imaging with indocyanine green. Jornal Brasileiro de Pneumologia. 2019;**45**(4):e20180401

[31] Chang TI, Chen YS, Huang SC. Intraoperative indocyanine green fluorescence lymphography to detect chylous leakage sites after congenital heart surgery. The Journal of Thoracic and Cardiovascular Surgery. 2014;**148**(2):739-740

[32] Kaburagi T, Takeuchi H, Oyama T, Nakamura R, Takahashi T, Wada N, et al. Intraoperative fluorescence lymphography using indocyanine green in a patient with chylothorax after esophagectomy: Report of a case. Surgery Today. 2013;**43**(2):206-210

[33] Pischik VG, Kovalenko A. The role of indocyanine green fluorescence for intersegmental plane identification during video-assisted thoracoscopic surgery segmentectomies. Journal of Thoracic Disease. 2018;**10**(Suppl. 31): S3704-S3711

[34] Wada H, Yamamoto T, Morimoto J, Sakairi Y, Suzuki H, Nakajima T, et al. Near-infrared-guided pulmonary Segmentectomy after endobronchial Indocyanine green injection. The Annals of Thoracic Surgery. 2020;**109**(2):396-403

[35] Yuasa Y, Seike J, Yoshida T, Takechi H, Yamai H, Yamamoto Y, et al. Sentinel lymph node biopsy using intraoperative indocyanine green fluorescence imaging navigated with preoperative CT lymphography for superficial esophageal cancer. Annals of Surgical Oncology. 2012;**19**(2):486-493

[36] Schlottmann F, Barbetta A, Mungo B, Lidor AO, Molena D. Identification of the lymphatic drainage pattern of esophageal cancer with near-infrared fluorescent imaging. Journal of Laparoendoscopic & Advanced Surgical Techniques. Part A. 2017;**27**(3):268-271

[37] Hachey KJ, Gilmore DM, Armstrong KW, Harris SE, Hornick JL, Colson YL, et al. Safety and feasibility of near-infrared image-guided lymphatic mapping of regional lymph nodes in esophageal cancer. The Journal of Thoracic and Cardiovascular Surgery. 2016;**152**(2):546-554

[38] Kim HK, Quan YH, Oh Y, Park JY, Park JH, Choi Y, et al. Macrophage-targeted Indocyanine green-Neomannosyl human serum albumin for intraoperative sentinel lymph node mapping in porcine esophagus. The Annals of Thoracic Surgery. 2016;**102**(4):1149-1155

[39] van Hagen P, Hulshof MCCM, van Lanschot JJB, Steyerberg EW, van Berge

Henegouwen MI, Wijnhoven BPL, et al. Preoperative chemoradiotherapy for esophageal or junctional cancer. The New England Journal of Medicine. 2012;**366**(22):2074-2084

[40] Karliczek A, Harlaar NJ, Zeebregts CJ, Wiggers T, Baas PC, van Dam GM. Surgeons lack predictive accuracy for anastomotic leakage in gastrointestinal surgery. International Journal of Colorectal Disease. 2009;**24**(5):569-576

[41] Slooter MD, Eshuis WJ, Cuesta MA, Gisbertz SS, van Berge Henegouwen MI. Fluorescent imaging using indocyanine green during esophagectomy to prevent surgical morbidity: A systematic review and meta-analysis. Journal of Thoracic Disease. 2019;**11**(Suppl 5):S755-S765

[42] Degett TH, Andersen HS, Gögenur I. Indocyanine green fluorescence angiography for intraoperative assessment of gastrointestinal anastomotic perfusion: A systematic review of clinical trials. Langenbeck's Archives of Surgery. 2016;**401**(6):767-775

[43] Ishige F, Nabeya Y, Hoshino I, Takayama W, Chiba S, Arimitsu H, et al. Quantitative assessment of the blood perfusion of the gastric conduit by Indocyanine green imaging. The Journal of Surgical Research. 2019;**234**:303-310

[44] Yukaya T, Saeki H, Kasagi Y, Nakashima Y, Ando K, Imamura Y, et al. Indocyanine green fluorescence angiography for quantitative evaluation of gastric tube perfusion in patients undergoing Esophagectomy. Journal of the American College of Surgeons. 2015;**221**(2):e37-e42

[45] Koyanagi K, Ozawa S, Oguma J, Kazuno A, Yamazaki Y, Ninomiya Y, et al. Blood flow speed of the gastric conduit assessed by indocyanine green fluorescence: New predictive evaluation of anastomotic leakage after esophagectomy. Medicine (Baltimore). 2016;**95**(30):e4386

[46] Kumagai Y, Hatano S, Sobajima J, Ishiguro T, Fukuchi M, Ishibashi KI, et al. Indocyanine green fluorescence angiography of the reconstructed gastric tube during esophagectomy: Efficacy of the 90-second rule. Diseases of the Esophagus: Official Journal of International Society Diseases of the Esophagus. 2018;**31**(12). DOI: 10.1093/dote/doy052. PMID: 29897432

[47] Slooter MD, de Bruin DM, Eshuis WJ, Veelo DP, van Dieren S, Gisbertz SS, et al. Quantitative fluorescence-guided perfusion assessment of the gastric conduit to predict anastomotic complications after esophagectomy. Diseases of the Esophagus: Official Journal of International Society Diseases of the Esophagus. 2021;**34**(5):doaa100

[48] Nakashima Y, Saeki H, Yukaya T, Tsutsumi S, Nakanishi R, Sugiyama M, et al. Blood flow assessment with Indocyanine green fluorescence angiography for Pedicled omental flap on cervical Esophagogastric anastomosis after Esophagectomy. Journal of the American College of Surgeons. 2016;**222**(5):e67-e69

Chapter 3

# Upper Gastrointestinal Endoscopy for Screening or Surveillance: Complication Avoidance and a Closer Look at the Esophagus

*Jihwan Ko*


## Abstract

Upper gastrointestinal endoscopy is the most important test used to diagnose esophageal disease. Proper insertion of the endoscope is essential for accurate examination of the esophagus. However, due to coughing or the gag reflex, esophageal examinations can be difficult. Further, when a central ridge is present in the middle of the pyriform sinus, careful approach is necessary. Chromoendoscopy of the esophagus includes acetic acid chromoendoscopy for Barrett's esophagus and lugol's iodine chromoendoscopy for squamous cell carcinoma. In recent times, electronic chromoendoscopy is widely used. In this chapter, diagnosis and treatment of various esophageal diseases including esophagitis, Barrett's esophagus, adenocarcinoma, squamous cell carcinoma, diverticulum, inlet patch, hiatal hernia, polyps, subepithelial lesions, and varix are discussed.


**Keywords:** gastrointestinal endoscope, cancer screening, esophageal disease, esophageal cancer, diagnosis

## 1. Introduction

Upper gastrointestinal endoscopy is the most important test for the diagnosis of esophageal disease. Accurate diagnosis is crucial for appropriate treatment of esophageal diseases, including surgical intervention. With advancements in the surgical treatment of esophageal diseases, the importance of upper gastrointestinal endoscopy has been increasing. In this chapter, the endoscopic techniques used in the examination of the esophagus are discussed.

## 2. Insertion technique

During endoscope insertion, the cough or gag reflex is induced and the movement of the esophageal lumen increases, thereby making esophageal examination difficult. Therefore, proper endoscope insertion is essential for accurate examination of the esophagus.

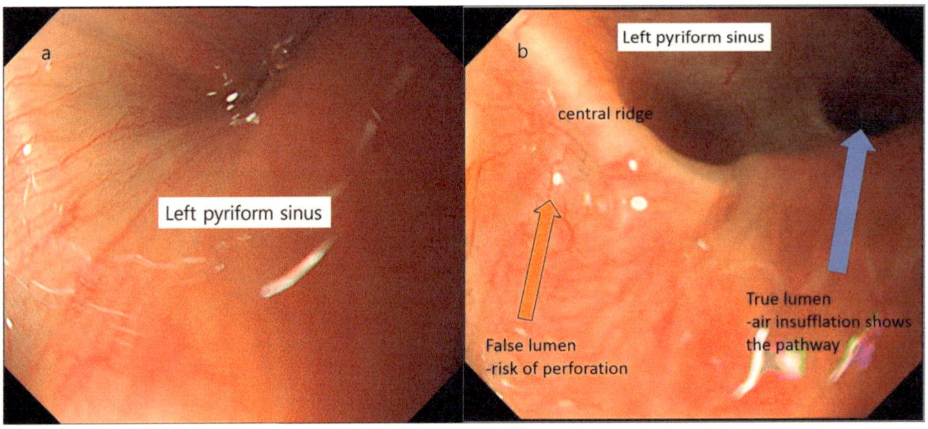


**Figure 1.**
*Two types of pyriform sinus. (a) Left pyriform sinus without central ridge. (b) Left pyriform sinus with central ridge.*

The first obstacle encountered during endoscope insertion is the uvula. Access to the pyriform sinus can be gained without difficulty if the endoscope is carefully inserted to the right or left of the uvula, taking care not to make contact with the centrally placed uvula. The second and most difficult part of endoscope insertion is the insertion of the endoscope into the pyriform sinus. This part is sometimes problematic for beginners, as well as for board-certified endoscopists. Upon reaching the left pyriform sinus, a slight clockwise rotation of the scope with gentle pressure is recommended for insertion in the left pyriform sinus [1]. This technique is successful in most cases; however, in some patients with anatomical variations, endoscopists experience severe resistance that may lead to bleeding or even perforation. Two types of pyriform sinus are shown in **Figure 1**. In **Figure 1a**, there is no central ridge; thus, the clockwise rotation technique can be used. In contrast, in **Figure 1b**, a central ridge is present in the left pyriform sinus, and the true lumen is more medial than normal, but its path runs upward (i.e., medially). After traversing the pyriform sinus, the path goes downward (i.e., laterally). Thus, performing the clockwise rotation technique without checking for the central ridge can result in severe pyriform sinus injury. Further, air insufflation is needed to determine the presence of a central ridge.

## 3. Chromoendoscopy

Chromoendoscopy entails the application of a chemical substance to the mucosal surface of the gastrointestinal tract to facilitate visualization and detection of dysplastic and malignant lesions [2]. Since the recent introduction and adoption of virtual chromoendoscopy methods such as narrow-band imaging (NBI), the importance of dye-based chromoendoscopy in day-to-day clinical practice has been decreasing [3]. Nevertheless, chromoendoscopy remains important in many clinical conditions. In this chapter, some chromoendoscopy methods still used in esophageal endoscopy will be discussed.

### 3.1 Acetic acid chromoendoscopy for Barrett's esophagus (BE)

Acetic acid is a weak acid that breaks up the disulfide bridges of glycoproteins of the mucus layer, resulting in protein denaturation and surface pattern enhancement [2]. BE is a known risk factor of high-grade dysplasia (HGD) and esophageal adenocarcinoma (EAC). Current nondysplastic BE surveillance guidelines recommend that random four-quadrant biopsy specimens be taken every 1–2 cm to check for dysplasia [4]. Due to the time-consuming and labor-intensive nature of the procedure, the American Society for Gastrointestinal Endoscopy Technology Committee released the Preservation and Incorporation of Valuable endoscopic Innovations (PIVI) criteria for nondysplastic BE surveillance. These criteria help determine which advanced imaging technique with targeted biopsy can replace the current surveillance guidelines for the detection of HGD and EAC. The performance thresholds in the PIVI criteria are per-patient sensitivity ≥90%, negative predictive value ≥98%, and specificity ≥80% [1]. Based on these criteria, only acetic acid chromoendoscopy, NBI, and confocal laser endomicroscopy can replace the current guidelines [4]. However, the use of acetic acid chromoendoscopy is on the decline due to the long procedural time, uneven distribution of dye over the mucosa, and high interobserver variability due to lack of classification [5].

### 3.2 Lugol's iodine chromoendoscopy

Lugol solution is an iodine-based solution used in the detection of dysplasia and cancer in squamous epithelia. Since iodine binds to glycogen, which is abundant in nonkeratinized squamous epithelium, and neoplastic tissues have low glycogen levels, they are not stained by Lugol solution [2]. Lugol staining has long been regarded as the gold standard for the detection and delineation of squamous cell carcinoma (SCC) and squamous dysplasia [6]. However, Lugol solution can cause thyrotoxicosis in patients with thyroid disease, iodine hypersensitivity, and retrosternal discomfort [2]. Regarding the avoidance of these side effects, several studies have compared Lugol's iodine chromoendoscopy and NBI. A recent meta-analysis revealed no significant difference in diagnostic sensitivity between the two methods (88% versus 92%); it also revealed that NBI has a significantly higher specificity than Lugol's iodine chromoendoscopy (88% versus 82%) [7]. Furthermore, several observational studies reported no significant difference in complete resection rate between the two methods [8, 9].

## 4. Electronic chromoendoscopy

Electronic chromoendoscopy involves endoscopic imaging technologies that provide detailed contrast enhancement of the mucosal surface and blood vessels in the form of electronic signals that can be analyzed using various image-processing techniques [10, 11]. There are various types of electronic chromoendoscopy, and they include NBI, i-SCAN, and flexible spectral imaging color enhancement (FICE).

### 4.1 NBI

NBI is an endoscopic optical image enhancement technology based on the penetration properties of light. An NBI filter in front of a xenon arc lamp produces two narrow bands of light with wavelengths of 415 nm and 540 nm [10]. Capillaries in the superficial mucosa are highlighted by the 415-nm-wavelength light band and appear brown. The longer 540-nm-wavelength light band makes deeper-lying veins appear blue-green [11]. Due to an abundance of blood vessels in the submucosal layer, a normal esophagus appears pale green on NBI [12]. Thus, lesions can be observed in great detail as a result of the color contrast effect at the mucosa of the gastroesophageal junction (GEJ) and in cases of early esophageal SCC (ESCC) [11].

### 4.2 i-SCAN

i-SCAN (Pentax, Tokyo, Japan) is another postprocessing digital contrast technology that consists of three enhancement features: surface enhancement, which sharpens the image; contrast enhancement, where darker (depressed) areas look bluer; and tone enhancement, a form of digital narrowed-spectrum imaging [13]. It was reported in several studies that i-SCAN is superior to white-light endoscopy (WLE) in the detection of reflux esophagitis and dysplasia in BE [14, 15]. However, i-SCAN is a relatively recent technology compared with NBI, and further research is still needed.

### 4.3 FICE

The FICE system takes an ordinary endoscopic image of different parts of the gastrointestinal mucosa from the video processor and arithmetically processes and estimates it to produce an image of a given dedicated wavelength between 400 and 700 nm. Single-wavelength images are randomly selected and assigned the colors red, green, and blue to build and display virtually enhanced color images [16]. A previous study compared WLE and the FICE system for the diagnosis of BE, but additional research is needed [17].

## 5. Artificial intelligence (AI)

In this section, understanding of the concepts of AI, machine learning (ML), deep learning (DL), and convolutional neural network (CNN) is essential. AI is the broadest term used in the description of machines that mimic human intelligence [18]. ML is a subfield of AI, and DL is a subfield of ML. ML is divided into supervised learning and unsupervised learning. In supervised learning, labeled datasets are used to train algorithms to classify data or predict outcomes accurately. In contrast, in unsupervised learning, unlabeled datasets are used to train algorithms [19]. In DL, unsupervised learning and neural networks are used. CNN is a type of artificial neural network used in image recognition and processing that is specifically designed to process pixel data [20]. AI is extensively used or studied with regard to the esophagus and will be considered at the end of the discussion of each disease.

## 6. Esophagitis

Esophagitis refers to inflammation or injury to the esophageal mucosa [21]. The types of esophagitis based on etiology include reflux esophagitis, infectious esophagitis, exfoliative esophagitis, eosinophilic esophagitis (EoE), and pill-induced esophagitis.

### 6.1 Reflux esophagitis

Gastroesophageal reflux disease (GERD) is a condition in which stomach contents reflux into the esophagus or beyond (e.g., into the oral cavity, larynx, or lungs) causing troublesome symptoms and complications [22]. The extent of mucosal breaks due to erosion or ulceration is the sole determinant of severity grade [23]. Grade A refers to one or more mucosal breaks no longer than 5 mm that do not extend beyond two mucosal folds. Grade B refers to one or more mucosal breaks more than 5 mm long that do not extend beyond two mucosal folds. Grade C refers to one or more mucosal breaks that extend beyond two or more mucosal folds but involve less than 75% of the esophageal circumference. Grade D refers to one or more mucosal breaks that involve at least 75% of the esophageal circumference. Currently, due to lack of interobserver agreement, minimal changes are not included in the GERD Los Angeles (LA) classification [23]. Recently, a DL model that uses CNNs for automatic classification and interpretation of routine GERD LA grades was proposed [24]. However, given that the available data are limited, more studies are needed.

### 6.2 Candida esophagitis

Esophageal candidiasis is the most common type of infectious esophagitis [25]. Immunocompromised patients are most at risk, and the most common symptoms are odynophagia, dysphagia, and retrosternal pain. Endoscopic examination is the best approach to diagnosing esophageal candidiasis, and multiple white plaques adherent to the mucosa are considered definitively diagnostic of the disease (**Figure 2**). The most common treatment is systemic and oral administration of fluconazole, an antifungal agent [25].

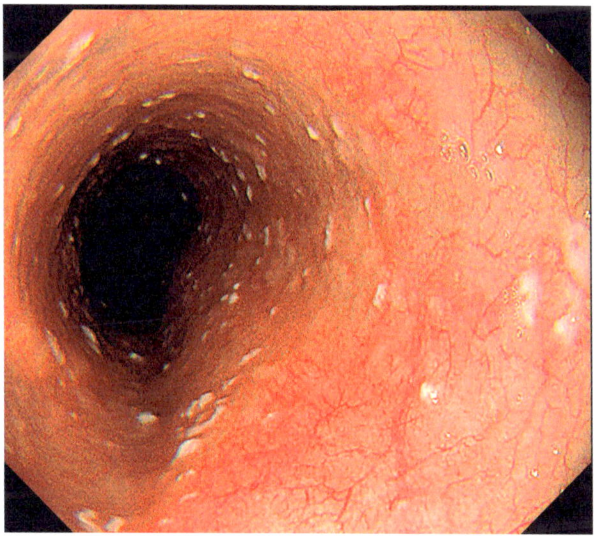

**Figure 2.**
*Esophageal candidiasis.*

### 6.3 Viral esophagitis

The two most common causes of viral esophagitis are herpes simplex virus (HSV) and cytomegalovirus (CMV). HSV esophagitis ulcers are circumscribed ulcers with raised edges that are described as volcano-like ulcers [26]. CMV esophagitis ulcers are well-demarcated vertical or horizontal linear shallow ulcers that occur in the middle and distal portions of the esophagus [27]. It is sometimes difficult to differentiate between HSV esophagitis and CMV esophagitis because their endoscopic characteristics often overlap [28]. Recently, an ML model for differentiating CMV esophagitis from HSV esophagitis was developed. It was developed based on the analysis of 87 patients with HSV esophagitis and 63 patients with CMV esophagitis using 666 endoscopic images of HSV esophagitis and 416 endoscopic images of CMV esophagitis. The sensitivity and specificity of the model were 100% [28].

### 6.4 Sloughing (exfoliative) esophagitis

Sloughing esophagitis is characterized by superficial necrotic squamous epithelium and endoscopic plaques or membranes (**Figure 3**) [29]. The symptoms include dysphagia, odynophagia, nausea, vomiting, abdominal pain, heartburn, chest pain, hematemesis, and obstructive symptoms secondary to the accumulation of casts in the esophageal lumen [30]. The pathogenesis is thought to involve exposure to drugs that cause esophageal damage or autoimmune conditions accompanied by esophageal damage. Such drugs include dabigatran, nonsteroidal anti-inflammatory drugs, bisphosphonates, and iron. The autoimmune conditions include celiac disease, pemphigus vulgaris, bullous pemphigoid, and lupus [30]. Prognosis is usually favorable, and long-term complications are rare. Treatment includes discontinuation of the offending agent and administration of proton-pump inhibitors (PPIs). Steroids may be helpful when a patient has an autoimmune condition [30].

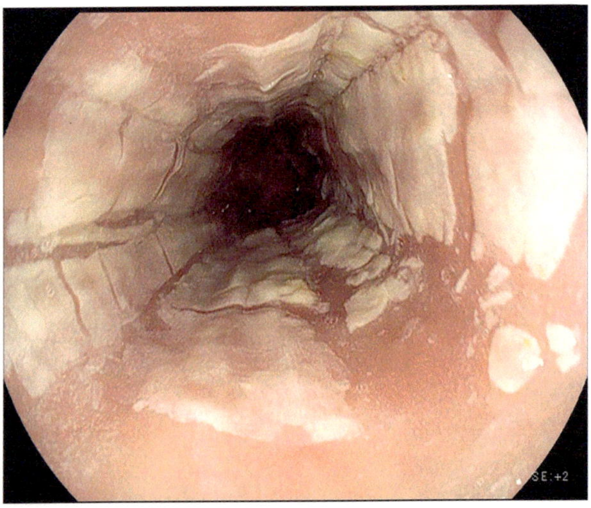


**Figure 3.**
*Sloughing esophagitis.*

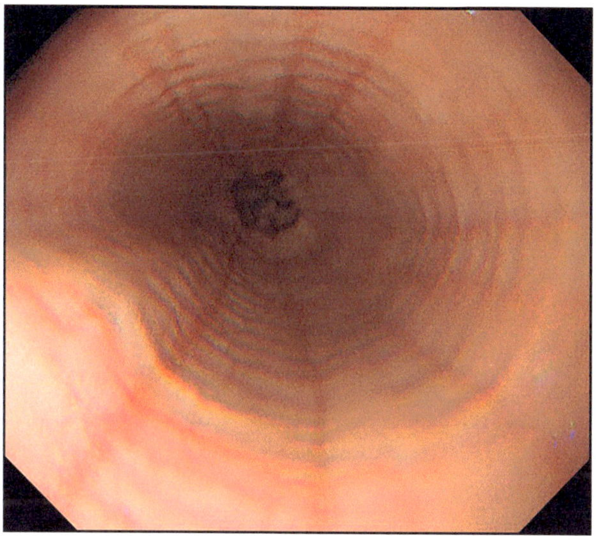

**Figure 4.**
*Eosinophilic esophagitis.*

### 6.5 EoE

EoE is a chronic immune-mediated inflammatory condition of the esophagus. Its symptoms are mainly related to esophageal dysfunction and include vomiting, dysphagia, and feeding difficulties. Diagnosis of EoE requires endoscopy with biopsy. The endoscopic findings include furrows (i.e., vertical lines in the mucosa), concentric rings, white plaques, edema, and stricture (**Figure 4**). The American College of Gastroenterology (ACG) recommends a minimum of six biopsies. A finding of 15 or more eosinophils per high-power field in the maximally affected area is required for diagnosis [31]. The treatment options are PPIs, topical corticosteroids, and allergy testing–directed elimination diet. A previous study presented a graphical representation of a suggested management algorithm [32].

### 6.6 Pill-induced esophagitis

Pill-induced esophagitis may present as erosions, kissing ulcers, and multiple small areas of ulceration with bleeding mainly in the middle third of the esophagus [33]. Treatment of pill-induced esophagitis consists of discontinuation of the offending drug and use of PPIs or sucralfate to hasten esophageal mucosal healing [34].

## 7. BE and early EAC

BE is a condition characterized by metaplasia of normal esophageal squamous epithelium to specialized columnar epithelium with goblet cells [35]. The ACG guidelines recommend considering BE when the length of the columnar mucosa is at least 1 cm. When BE is suspected, at least eight random biopsy samples should be taken if the BE segment length is <2 cm, and in patients with suspected long-segment BE, four biopsy samples should be taken for every 2 cm of BE segment [36]. Based on the length of

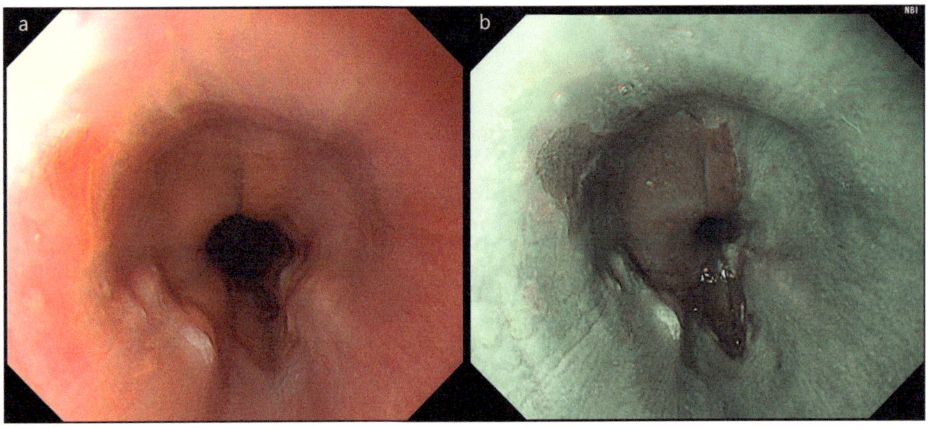


**Figure 5.**
*Barrett's esophagus. (a) WLE. (b) NBI.*

salmon-colored mucosa proximal to the GEJ, BE is classified into two groups: short-segment BE and long-segment BE (**Figure 5**). Long-segment BE is defined as BE with segment length ≥ 3 cm, and short-segment BE is defined as BE with segment length < 3 cm [36]. Screening endoscopy is recommended for patients with chronic GERD symptoms and three or more additional risk factors of BE (e.g., male gender, age > 50 years, white race, tobacco smoking, obesity, and history of BE or EAC in a first-degree relative) [35]. If screening endoscopy does not reveal dysplasia, surveillance endoscopy should be repeated in 3–5 years. Further, a histological grade of "indefinite for dysplasia" should be confirmed by a second pathologist with gastrointestinal expertise, PPI therapy should be initiated, and endoscopic biopsy should be repeated within 6 months [35]. When the histological grade is low-grade dysplasia (LGD), endoscopic mucosal resection or endoscopic submucosal dissection of all visible lesions should be performed, followed by ablation of the remaining BE segment (i.e., endoscopic eradication therapy [EET]) with the goal of complete eradication of intestinal metaplasia (CEIM). Alternatively, surveillance can be performed every 6 months for the first year and annually thereafter [36]. When the histological grade is HGD or intramucosal carcinoma (T1a), EET with the goal of CEIM should be performed. It is recommended to enroll patients with LGD or HGD for surveillance and reflux control after CEIM is achieved [35]. Surveillance at 1 year after CEIM and every 2 years thereafter is recommended for patients with LGD. Surveillance at 3, 6, and 12 months after CEIM and annually thereafter is recommended for patients with HGD or intramucosal carcinoma [35]. Esophagectomy is typically recommended for patients with EAC and submucosal invasion (T1b). Alternatively, EET can be considered for patients with superficial submucosal invasion (sm1, to a depth < 500 μm) and low-risk features such as negative deep margin, well-moderate differentiation, and absence of lymphovascular invasion [35]. Regarding neoplasia detection, the sensitivity and specificity of AI are >90% and > 80%, respectively. Further, regarding neoplasia characterization, the sensitivity and specificity of AI are 90% and 88%, respectively [37].

## 8. ESCC

ESCC is the most common type of esophageal cancer worldwide; it is especially common in Asia and Africa (**Figure 6**) [38]. The risk factors for ESCC include

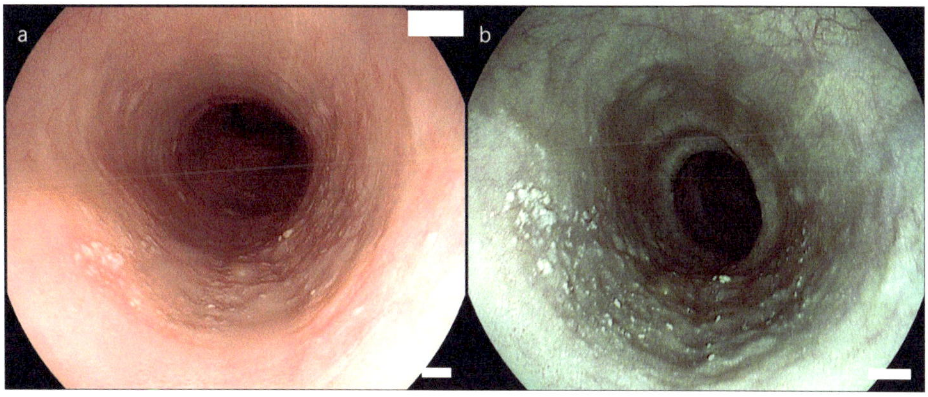


**Figure 6.**
*Esophageal squamous cell carcinoma. (a) WLE, (b) tone enhancement mode with i-scan.*

long-standing exposure to tobacco and alcohol, achalasia, head and neck squamous cell cancer, tylosis, history of lye ingestion, celiac sprue, and hot liquid ingestion [39]. In addition, the etiological role of human papilloma virus infection is under study [39]. Endoscopic screening should be considered in the presence of risk factors. Infiltration depth prediction is important since it is primarily associated with lymph node metastasis [40]. The Japan Esophageal Society uses a simplified classification of vessel irregularities known as intrapapillary capillary loops (IPCLs) to predict infiltration depth. Type A vessel refers to a normal or abnormal microvessel without severe irregularity, that is, a microvessel with normal epithelium or inflammation and low-grade intraepithelial neoplasia [41]. Abnormal microvessels with severe irregularity or highly dilated abnormal vessels are classified as type B1, B2, or B3. Type B1 vessels have loop-like formations and a predicted invasion depth of epithelium (EP) or lamina propria mucosae (LMP). Type B2 vessels do not have loop-like formations, and their predicted invasion depth is muscularis mucosae or submucosa (SM1). Type B3 vessels have highly dilated vessels and a predicted invasion depth of the submucosa (SM2) or deeper [41]. ESD is recommended for lesions with invasion depth of T1a-EP/T1a-LMP, noncircumferential lesions, and circumferential lesions with lengths ≤5 cm. Furthermore, ESD can be used to remove noncircumferential lesions with invasion depth of T1a-MM/T1b-SM1. Surgery or chemoradiation should be considered when the invasion depth is T1a-EP/T1a-LMP and lateral extension is circumferential with length > 5 cm. It should also be considered when the invasion depth is T1a-MM/T1b-SM1 and lateral extension is circumferential [39]. In a recent study by Everson et al., it was reported that the sensitivity and specificity of AI using CNN for the classification of abnormal IPCL patterns were 89.3% and 98%, respectively [42].

## 9. Esophageal diverticulum

Esophageal diverticula are a rare condition that causes dysphagia, regurgitation, and chest pain [43]. They are classified into two: pulsion diverticula and traction diverticula. Pulsion diverticula are associated with increased intraluminal pressure, which causes herniation. Zenker's diverticulum, which is a pulsion-type pharyngoesophageal pseudodiverticulum, is the most common type of esophageal diverticulum (**Figure 7**) [44]. Surgery can be considered for the management of Zenker's

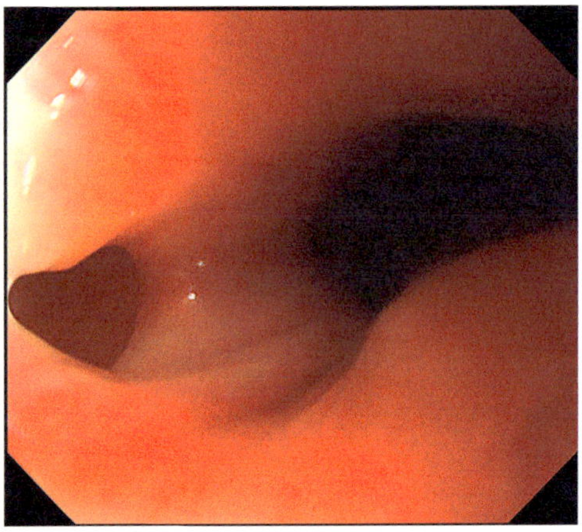

**Figure 7.**
*Zenker's diverticulum.*

diverticulum. However, the current first-line treatment involves cutting the entire septum and creating a common cavity between the esophagus and the diverticulum [45]. There are two methods of endoscopic septum division. The first is conventional flexible endoscopic septum division, which entails full-thickness incision of the mucosa, submucosa, and the muscular fibers to create a common cavity between the esophagus and the diverticulum. The second is Zenker's diverticulum per-oral endoscopic myotomy, which entails minimal mucosal incision to advance the endoscope into the submucosal space of the septum. Complete septotomy is then performed, and the mucosal incision site is securely closed with several endoclips [45].

## 10. Esophageal inlet patch

Esophageal inlet patches (IPs) are well-circumscribed areas of mucosa that are salmon-pink in color, variable in size, and oval-round or even geographically shaped (**Figure 8**) [46]. Most IPs are located just below the upper esophageal sphincter or in the postcricoid region of the esophagus [46]. Since most IPs present with no symptoms and are located in the upper esophagus, where endoscopists tend to pass the

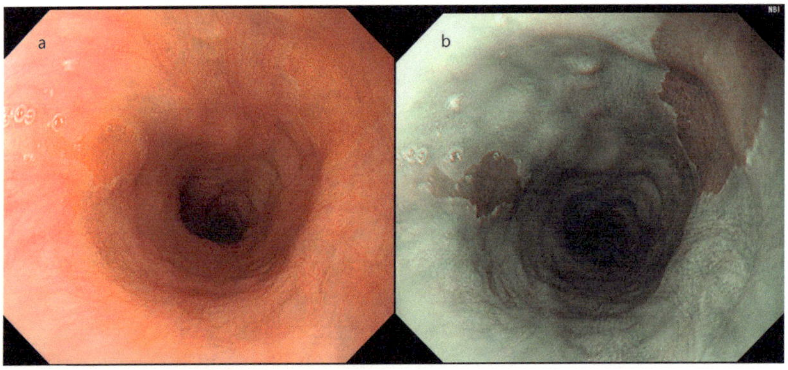


**Figure 8.**
*Esophageal inlet patch. (a) WLE. (b) NBI.*

endoscope quickly, it is difficult to identify and observe IPs in detail. However, since adenocarcinomas sometimes arise in IPs, careful observation is necessary [47]. It is recommended that WLE be used first when inserting the endoscope and NBI be used to observe the esophagus up to the pyriform sinus when retracting the endoscope.

## 11. Esophageal stricture

Esophageal stricture is an abnormal narrowing of the esophageal lumen (**Figure 9**). It can be benign or malignant. The etiology of benign esophageal stricture includes corrosive substance ingestion, EoE, radiation injury, and drug-induced esophagitis. Treatment includes mechanical or balloon dilation, esophageal stents, or surgical management [48].

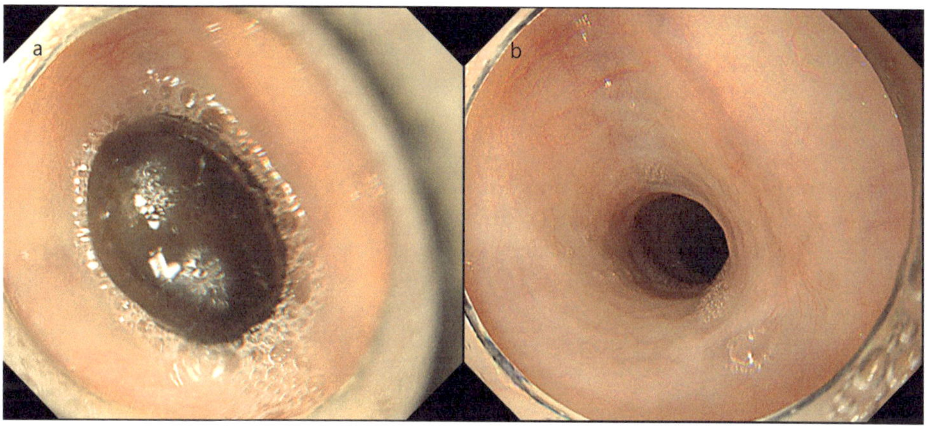


**Figure 9.**
*Esophageal stricture: (a) with a bean stuck in the stricture; (b) after bean removal.*

## 12. Esophageal hiatal hernia

Hiatal hernia is a condition in which the upper part of the stomach bulges through an aperture in the diaphragm (**Figure 10**). There are four anatomical classifications of hiatal hernia: types 1, 2, 3, and 4. Type 1 or sliding hernias are associated with symmetrical

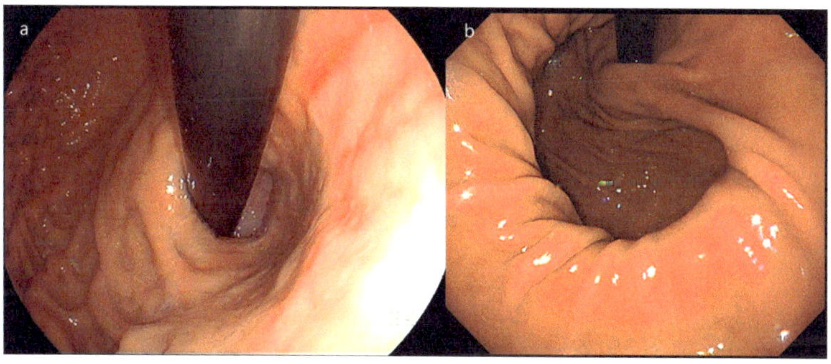


**Figure 10.**
*Esophageal hiatal hernia: (a) sliding-type hiatal hernia; (b) paraesophageal hernia (mixed type).*

ascent of the stomach through the diaphragmatic crus. A patient with type 1 hernia who has reflux symptoms can first undergo PPI therapy with lifestyle modification. In contrast, a patient with symptomatic paraesophageal hernia (types 2, 3, and 4) is at high risk for obstruction, and surgery should be considered for such a patient [49].

## 13. Esophageal polyps

### 13.1 Esophageal squamous papilloma

Esophageal squamous papilloma is a wart-like exophytic mass located in the middle to distal esophagus (**Figure 11**). Most papillomas are benign, small, and can be easily removed during forceps biopsy. However, owing to the few reported cases of carcinomatous transformation of these lesions, definite removal is necessary if a papilloma bleeds, is unusually large, elicits foreign-body sensation, or shows atypical changes on histological examination [50].

### 13.2 Sentinel polyp

Esophageal sentinel polyps (or sentinel folds) are inflammatory polyps at the GEJ associated with recurrent GERD (**Figure 12**) [51]. Although sentinel polyps are benign, biopsy is indicated if a lesion is discovered for the first time or if it changes in size or shape.

### 13.3 Hyperplastic polyp

Hyperplastic polyps are uncommon lesions that most commonly occur at the GEJ (**Figure 13**) [52]. There are no reported cases of malignant transformation of esophageal hyperplastic polyps [52]. However, when the polyp size is larger than 10 mm, it is

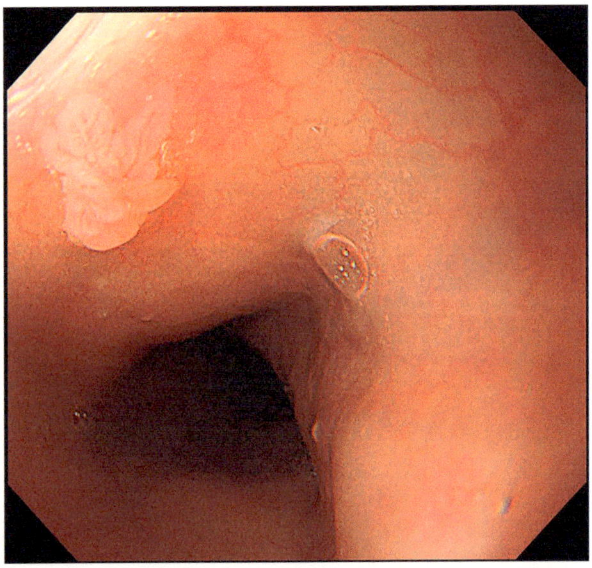

**Figure 11.**
*Esophageal squamous papilloma.*

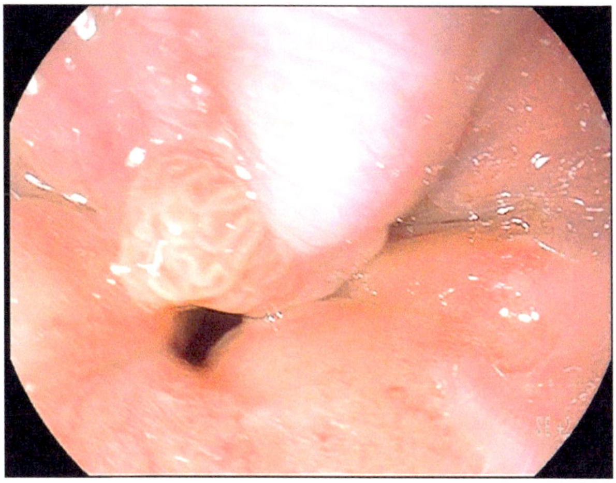

**Figure 12.**
*Sentinel polyp.*

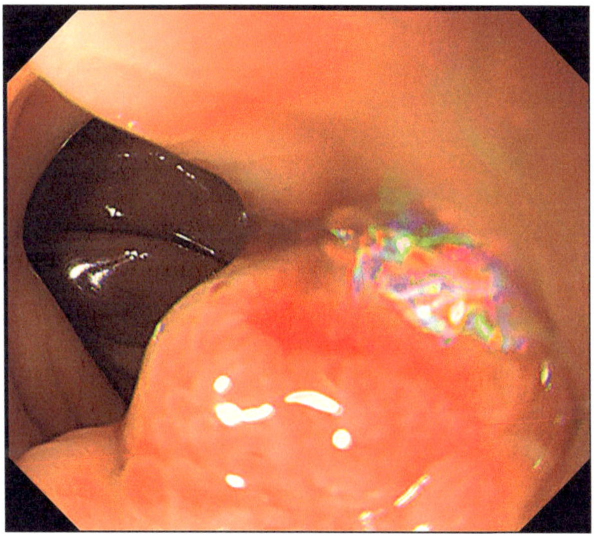

**Figure 13.**
*Hyperplastic polyp at the GEJ.*

difficult to determine if the polyp originated from the GEJ or from the gastric cardia; in such cases, complete removal of the polyp should be considered [53].

## 14. Esophageal subepithelial lesions

Subepithelial lesions (SELs) of the gastrointestinal tract are tumors that originate from the muscularis mucosa, submucosa, or muscularis propria [54]. The most common (70–80%) benign esophageal SEL is leiomyoma [55]. However, carcinoid tumors, lymphomas, glomus tumors, and gastrointestinal stromal tumors (GISTs) are malignant or have malignant potential and must be considered [56]. The 2022 European

Society of Gastrointestinal Endoscopy (ESGE) guidelines do not recommend WLE or advanced imaging techniques for the characterization of SEL subtypes. Furthermore, the guidelines recommend endoscopic ultrasonography (EUS) as the best tool for the characterization of features of SEL (e.g., size, location, originating layer, echogenicity, shape), but EUS alone cannot distinguish between the types of SEL. Tissue diagnosis is required for SELs with features suggestive of GIST, size >20 mm, high-risk stigmata, or requirement of surgical resection or oncological treatment. The ESGE suggests esophagogastroduodenoscopy (EGD) surveillance at 3–6 months if asymptomatic SELs are found on EGD. EGD is recommended at intervals of 2–3 years for lesions <10 mm and at intervals of 1–2 years for lesions 10–20 mm in size. For asymptomatic unresected SELs >20 mm in size, the ESGE recommends surveillance with EGD plus EUS at 6 months, and then at intervals of 6–12 months [54].

## 15. Esophageal varix on screening and surveillance

Esophageal varices are dilated submucosal veins of the distal esophagus that connect the portal and systemic circulations (**Figure 14**) [57]. General rules for describing endoscopic findings of esophageal varix were proposed by the Japan Society for Portal Hypertension [58]. The rules define six main categories: location (L), form (F), color (C), red color (RC) signs, bleeding signs, and mucosal findings. Regarding location, Ls, Lm, and Li stand for Locus superior, Locus medialis, and Locus inferior, respectively. Regarding form, F0 denotes no varicose appearance, F1 denotes straight small-caliber varices, F2 denotes moderately enlarged and beady varices, and F3 denotes markedly enlarged, nodular, or tumor-shaped varices. Regarding color, Cw denotes white varices, Cb denotes blue varices, CwTh denotes thrombosed white varices, and Cb-Th denotes thrombosed blue varices. Regarding RC signs, RWM denotes red wale markings, CRS denotes cherry red spots, HCS denotes hematocystic spots, and Te denotes telangiectasia. Nonselective beta-blockers (e.g., nadolol, propranolol, carvedilol) should be considered if small ($\leq$5 mm) varices with RWM or medium/large (>5 mm) varices are found on screening endoscopy [59].

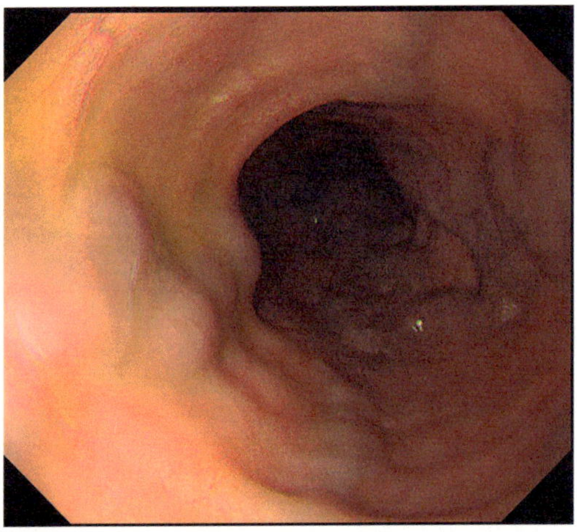

**Figure 14.**
*Esophageal varix.*

## Conflict of interest

The authors declare no conflict of interest.

## Author details

Jihwan Ko
Baekyang Jeil Internal Medicine Clinic, Busan, South Korea

*Address all correspondence to: jihwanko65@gmail.com

## References


[1] Park KS. Introduction to starting upper gastrointestinal endoscopy: Proper insertion, complete observation, and appropriate photographing. Clinical Endoscopy. 2015;**48**:279-284. DOI: 10.5946/ce.2015.48.4.279

[2] Trivedi PJ, Braden B. Indications, stains and techniques in chromoendoscopy. QJM. 2013;**106**: 117-131. DOI: 10.1093/qjmed/hcs186

[3] Singh R, Chiam KH, Leiria F, Pu LZCT, Choi KC, Militz M. Chromoendoscopy: Role in modern endoscopic imaging. Translational Gastroenterology and Hepatology. 2020;**5**:39. DOI: 10.21037/tgh.2019.12.06

[4] ASGE Technology Committee, Thosani N, Abu Dayyeh BK, Sharma P, Aslanian HR, Enestvedt BK, et al. ASGE technology committee systematic review and meta-analysis assessing the ASGE preservation and incorporation of valuable endoscopic innovations thresholds for adopting real-time imaging-assisted endoscopic targeted biopsy during endoscopic surveillance of Barrett's esophagus. Gastrointestinal Endoscopy. 2016;**83**:684-698.e7. DOI: 10.1016/j.gie.2016.01.007

[5] Sanghi V, Thota PN. Barrett's esophagus: Novel strategies for screening and surveillance. Therapeutic Advances in Chronic Disease. 2019;**10**:2040622319837851. DOI: 10.1177/2040622319837851

[6] Barret M, Prat F. Diagnosis and treatment of superficial esophageal cancer. Annals of Gastroenterology. 2018;**31**:256-265. DOI: 10.20524/aog.2018.0252

[7] Morita FH, Bernardo WM, Ide E, Rocha RS, Aquino JC, Minata MK, et al. Narrow band imaging versus lugol chromoendoscopy to diagnose squamous cell carcinoma of the esophagus: A systematic review and meta-analysis. BMC Cancer. 2017;**17**:54. DOI: 10.1186/s12885-016-3011-9

[8] Costa-Santos MP, Ferreira AO, Mouradides C, Pérez-Cuadrado-Robles E, Yeung R, Garcés-Duran R, et al. Is Lugol necessary for endoscopic resection of esophageal squamous cell neoplasia? Endoscopy International Open. 2020;**8**:E1471-E1477. DOI: 10.1055/a-1198-4316

[9] Li J, Shen X, Geng Y, Chen J, Shi X, Liu F, et al. Demarcation of early esophageal squamous cell carcinoma during endoscopic submucosal dissection: A comparison study between Lugol's iodine staining and narrow-band imaging. Medicine. 2021;**100**:e27760. DOI: 10.1097/MD.0000000000027760

[10] ASGE Technology Committee, Manfredi MA, Abu Dayyeh BK, Bhat YM, Chauhan SS, Gottlieb KT, et al. Electronic chromoendoscopy. Gastrointestinal Endoscopy. 2015;**81**: 249-261. DOI: 10.1016/j.gie.2014.06.020

[11] Jang JY. The past, present, and future of image-enhanced endoscopy. Clinical Endoscopy. 2015;**48**:466-475. DOI: 10.5946/ce.2015.48.6.466

[12] Cho WY, Jang JY, Lee DH. Recent advances in image-enhanced endoscopy. Clinical Endoscopy. 2011;**44**:65-75. DOI: 10.5946/ce.2011.44.2.65

[13] East JE, Vleugels JL, Roelandt P, Bhandari P, Bisschops R, Dekker E, et al. Advanced endoscopic imaging: European Society of Gastrointestinal Endoscopy (ESGE) technology review.

Endoscopy. 2016;**48**:1029-1045. DOI: 10.1055/s-0042-118087

[14] Kang HS, Hong SN, Kim YS, Park HS, Kim BK, Lee JH, et al. The efficacy of i-SCAN for detecting reflux esophagitis: A prospective randomized controlled trial. Diseases of the Esophagus. 2013;**26**:204-211. DOI: 10.1111/j.1442-2050.2012.01427.x

[15] Hoffman A, Korczynski O, Tresch A, Hansen T, Rahman F, Goetz M, et al. Acetic acid compared with i-scan imaging for detecting Barrett's esophagus: A randomized, comparative trial. Gastrointestinal Endoscopy. 2014;**79**:46-54. DOI: 10.1016/j.gie.2013.07.013

[16] Cho JH. Advanced imaging technology other than narrow band imaging. Clinical Endoscopy. 2015;**48**:503-510. DOI: 10.5946/ce.2015.48.6.503

[17] Osawa H, Yamamoto H, Yamada N, Yoshizawa M, Sunada K, Kita H, et al. Diagnosis of endoscopic Barrett's esophagus by transnasal flexible spectral imaging color enhancement. Journal of Gastroenterology. 2009;**44**:1125-1132. DOI: 10.1007/s00535-009-0121-z

[18] AI Vs. Machine Learning Vs. Deep Learning Vs. Neural Networks: What's the Difference? 2020. Available from: https://www.ibm.com/cloud/blog/ai-vs-machine-learning-vs-deep-learning-vs-neural-networks [Accessed: April 22, 2022]

[19] Supervised Vs. Unsupervised Learning: What's the Difference? 2021. Available from: https://www.ibm.com/cloud/blog/supervised-vs-unsupervised-learning [Accessed: April 22, 2022]

[20] Convolutional Neural Network. 2018. Available from: https://www.techtarget.com/searchenterpriseai/definition/convolutional-neural-network [Accessed: April 22, 2022]

[21] Esophagitis. 2021. Available from: https://www.ncbi.nlm.nih.gov/books/NBK442012/ [Accessed: April 23, 2022]

[22] Reflux Esophagitis. 2021. Available from: https://www.ncbi.nlm.nih.gov/books/NBK554462/ [Accessed: April 23, 2022]

[23] LA Classification. 2022. Available from: https://iwgco.net/la-classification/ [Accessed: April 23, 2022]

[24] Wang CC, Chiu YC, Chen WL, Yang TW, Tsai MC, Tseng MH. A deep learning model for classification of endoscopic gastroesophageal reflux disease. International Journal of Environmental Research and Public Health. 2021;**18**:2428. DOI: 10.3390/ijerph18052428

[25] Mohamed AA, Lu XL, Mounmin FA. Diagnosis and treatment of esophageal candidiasis: Current updates. Canadian Journal of Gastroenterology & Hepatology. 2019;**2019**:3585136. DOI: 10.1155/2019/3585136

[26] Monsanto P, Almeida N, Cipriano MA, Gouveia H, Sofia C. Concomitant herpetic and eosinophilic esophagitis--a causality dilemma. Acta Gastroenterologica Belgica. 2012;**75**:361-363

[27] Marques S, Carmo J, Pinto D, Bispo M, Ramos S, Chagas C. Cytomegalovirus disease of the upper gastrointestinal tract: A 10-year retrospective study. GE Portuguese Journal of Gastroenterology. 2017;**24**:262-268. DOI: 10.1159/000479232

[28] Lee JS, Yun J, Ham S, Park H, Lee H, Kim J, et al. Machine learning approach for differentiating

cytomegalovirus esophagitis from herpes simplex virus esophagitis. Scientific Reports. 2021;**11**:3672. DOI: 10.1038/s41598-020-78556-z

[29] Purdy JK, Appelman HD, McKenna BJ. Sloughing esophagitis is associated with chronic debilitation and medications that injure the esophageal mucosa. Modern Pathology. 2012;**25**:767-775. DOI: 10.1038/modpathol.2011.204

[30] Then EO, Grantham T, Lopez M, Reddy M, Gaduputi V. Esophagitis dissecans superficialis (EDS) secondary to hair dye ingestion: Case report and literature review. Clinics and Practice. 2021;**11**:185-189. DOI: 10.3390/clinpract11020026

[31] Muir A, Falk GW. Eosinophilic esophagitis: A review. Journal of the American Medical Association. 2021;**326**:1310-1318. DOI: 10.1001/jama.2021.14920

[32] Gonsalves NP, Aceves SS. Diagnosis and treatment of eosinophilic esophagitis. The Journal of Allergy and Clinical Immunology. 2020;**145**:1-7. DOI: 10.1016/j.jaci.2019.11.011

[33] Abid S, Mumtaz K, Jafri W, Hamid S, Abbas Z, Shah HA, et al. Pill-induced esophageal injury: Endoscopic features and clinical outcomes. Endoscopy. 2005;**37**:740-744. DOI: 10.1055/s-2005-870129

[34] Zhang Y, Tong Y, Wang W, Xu L. Chest pain from pill-induced esophagitis: A rare side effect of ascorbic acid. SAGE Open Medical Case Reports. 10 May 2018;**6**:2050313X18775004. DOI: 10.1177/2050313X18775004

[35] Shaheen NJ, Falk GW, Iyer PG, Souza RF, Yadlapati RH, Sauer BG, et al. Diagnosis and management of Barrett's esophagus: An updated ACG guideline. The American Journal of Gastroenterology. 2022;**117**:559-587. DOI: 10.14309/ajg.0000000000001680

[36] Dam AN, Klapman J. A narrative review of Barrett's esophagus in 2020, molecular and clinical update. Annals of Translational Medicine. 2020;**8**:1107. DOI: 10.21037/atm-20-4406

[37] Hamade N, Sharma P. Artificial intelligence in Barrett's Esophagus. Therapeutic Advances in Gastrointestinal Endoscopy. 2021;**14**:26317745211049964. DOI: 10.1177/26317745211049964

[38] Codipilly DC, Qin Y, Dawsey SM, Kisiel J, Topazian M, Ahlquist D, et al. Screening for esophageal squamous cell carcinoma: Recent advances. Gastrointestinal Endoscopy. 2018;**88**:413-426. DOI: 10.1016/j.gie.2018.04.2352

[39] Esophageal Cancer Screening (PDQ®)-Health Professional Version. 2022. Available from: https://www.cancer.gov/types/esophageal/hp/esophageal-screening-pdq [Accessed: April 30, 2022]

[40] Dumoulin FL, Hildenbrand R, Oyama T, Steinbrück I. Current trends in endoscopic diagnosis and treatment of early esophageal cancer. Cancers (Basel). 2021;**13**:752. DOI: 10.3390/cancers13040752

[41] Oyama T, Inoue H, Arima M, Momma K, Omori T, Ishihara R, et al. Prediction of the invasion depth of superficial squamous cell carcinoma based on microvessel morphology: Magnifying endoscopic classification of the Japan Esophageal society. Esophagus. 2017;**14**:105-112. DOI: 10.1007/s10388-016-0527-7

[42] Everson M, Herrera L, Li W, Luengo IM, Ahmad O, Banks M, et al. Artificial intelligence for the real-time

classification of intrapapillary capillary loop patterns in the endoscopic diagnosis of early oesophageal squamous cell carcinoma: A proof-of-concept study. United European Gastroenterology Journal. 2019;7:297-306. DOI: 10.1177/2050640618821800

[43] Sato H, Takeuchi M, Hashimoto S, Mizuno KI, Furukawa K, Sato A, et al. Esophageal diverticulum: New perspectives in the era of minimally invasive endoscopic treatment. World Journal of Gastroenterology. 2019;**25**:1457-1464. DOI: 10.3748/wjg.v25.i12.1457

[44] Miutescu BP, Khan S, Mony S, Khashab MA. Role of peroral endoscopic myotomy (POEM) in the management of esophageal diverticula. Clinical Endoscopy. 2020;**53**:646-651. DOI: 10.5946/ce.2020.262

[45] Shimamura Y, Fujiyoshi MRA, Fujiyoshi Y, Nishikawa Y, Ono M, Owada K, et al. Per-oral endoscopic myotomy as treatment for Killian-Jamieson diverticulum. DEN Open. 2022;**2**:e27. DOI: 10.1002/deo2.27

[46] Ciocalteu A, Popa P, Ionescu M, Gheonea DI. Issues and controversies in esophageal inlet patch. World Journal of Gastroenterology. 2019;**25**:4061-4073. DOI: 10.3748/wjg.v25.i30.4061

[47] Tanaka M, Ushiku T, Ikemura M, Shibahara J, Seto Y, Fukayama M. Esophageal adenocarcinoma arising in cervical inlet patch with synchronous Barrett's esophagus-related dysplasia. Pathology International. 2014;**64**: 397-401. DOI: 10.1111/pin.12181

[48] Esophageal Stricture. 2021. Available from: https://www.ncbi.nlm.nih.gov/books/NBK542209/ [Accessed: May 7, 2022]

[49] Sfara A, Dumitrascu DL. The management of hiatal hernia: An update on diagnosis and treatment. Medicine and Pharmacy Reports. 2019;**92**:321-325. DOI: 10.15386/mpr-1323

[50] Cho JY, Cheung DY, Kim TJ, Kim JK. A case of esophageal squamous cell carcinoma in situ arising from esophageal squamous papilloma. Clinical Endoscopy. 2019;**52**:72-75. DOI: 10.5946/ce.2018.058

[51] Honda H, Kume K, Murakami H, Yamasaki T, Yoshikawa I, Otsuki M. Pseudomalignant erosion in hyperplastic polyp at esophago-gastric junction. Journal of Gastroenterology and Hepatology. 2005;**20**:800-801. DOI: 10.1111/j.1440-1746.2005.03210.x

[52] Tarar ZI, Tahan V, Yin F, Daglilar E. An unusual case of esophageal hyperplastic polyp with scleroderma: A case report and review of the literature. Cureus. 2021;**13**:e12500. DOI: 10.7759/cureus.12500

[53] Castro R, Pimentel-Nunes P, Dinis-Ribeiro M. Evaluation and management of gastric epithelial polyps. Best Practice & Research. Clinical Gastroenterology. 2017;**31**:381-387. DOI: 10.1016/j.bpg.2017.06.001

[54] Deprez PH, Moons LMG, O'Toole D, Gincul R, Seicean A, Pimentel-Nunes P, et al. Endoscopic management of subepithelial lesions including neuroendocrine neoplasms: European Society of Gastrointestinal Endoscopy (ESGE) guideline. Endoscopy. 2022;**54**:412-429. DOI: 10.1055/a-1751-5742

[55] Ko WJ, Song GW, Cho JY. Evaluation and endoscopic management of esophageal submucosal tumor. Clinical Endoscopy. 2017;**50**:250-253. DOI: 10.5946/ce.2016.109

[56] Cho JW, Korean ESD Study Group. Current guidelines in the management of upper gastrointestinal subepithelial tumors. Clinical Endoscopy. 2016;**49**: 235-240. DOI: 10.5946/ce.2015.096

[57] Esophageal Varices. 2021. Available from: https://www.ncbi.nlm.nih.gov/books/NBK448078/ [Accessed: May 8, 2022]

[58] Tajiri T, Yoshida H, Obara K, Onji M, Kage M, Kitano S, et al. General rules for recording endoscopic findings of esophagogastric varices (2nd edition). Digestive Endoscopy. 2010;**22**:1-9. DOI: 10.1111/j.1443-1661.2009.00929.x

[59] Garcia-Tsao G, Abraldes JG, Berzigotti A, Bosch J. Portal hypertensive bleeding in cirrhosis: Risk stratification, diagnosis, and management: 2016 practice guidance by the American association for the study of liver diseases. Hepatology. 2017;**65**:310-335. DOI: 10.1002/hep.28906

Section 2

# Benign Diseases

Chapter 4

# Perspective Chapter: Update on Achalasia Treatment

*Gad Marom, Ronit Brodie and Yoav Mintz*

## Abstract

Achalasia is a primary motility disorder of the esophagus characterized by failure of relaxation of the lower esophageal sphincter (LES) and aperistalsis of the esophagus. There are 3 types of achalasia, diagnosed and differentiated according to the Chicago classification using high resolution manometry (HRM). The classic symptoms of achalasia as described by the Eckardt score are dysphagia, retrosternal pain, regurgitation and weight loss. This chapter will discuss the interesting evolution of achalasia in the modern era, the ways to diagnose achalasia, different sub-groups within achalasia patients population, treat it with either endoscopic or surgical manner, pre-operative and post-operative considerations and routine follow-up.

**Keywords:** achalasia, Eckardt score, per-Oral endoscopic Myotomy, high resolution manometry, Endo-FLIP

## 1. Introduction

Achalasia is a primary motility disorder of the esophagus characterized by failure of relaxation of the lower esophageal sphincter (LES) and aperistalsis of the esophagus. There are 3 types of achalasia, diagnosed and differentiated according to the Chicago classification 4.0 using high resolution manometry (HRM) [1]. These types are differentiated by the functionality of the esophageal motility and do not reflect a progression of the disease from one to the other. The classic symptoms of achalasia include progressive dysphagia, retrosternal pain, regurgitation or vomiting of undigested food and weight loss [2].

Over the last few years, the incidence of achalasia has increased. Once thought to be a rare disease with an incidence of 0.03–1.63 per 100,000 persons per year, a higher incidence of 2.3–2.93 cases per 100,000 persons per year was recently reported [3, 4]. The upsurge in incidence may be attributed to the increased use of high-resolution manometry (HRM). This test has become more sensitive and easier to interpret due to better sensors and intuitive visualization of results. Additionally, the emergence of Per-Oral Endoscopic Myotomy (POEM) has also largely contributed to the increased of awareness of the disease.

The textbook presentation of patients with achalasia is outdated. Patients are no longer appearing as malnourished or cachectic as classically described [5, 6]. Counterintuitively, in recent years, due to the variety of calorie-rich, high fat soft and liquid foods, some achalasia patients have begun to present as overweight and even obese. These patients suffer from dysphagia and retrosternal pain but manage their symptoms via dietary changes and constant eating due to lack of satiety, which may further contribute to increased weight gain despite dysphagia. Additionally, the complaints of chest pain are often mistakenly contributed to a reflux disease that is more common among obese patients than achalasia, thereby delaying their diagnoses. It is quite common to find achalasia patients treated with antacid medications such as proton pump inhibitors, unsuccessfully, as the pathophysiology of achalasia is not rooted in acid reflux but regurgitation of undigested food.

Young achalasia patients often are misdiagnosed as suffering from eating disorders, specifically among adolescents and female gender [7, 8]. It is not uncommon for patients to be admitted to inpatient care for eating disorder, further delaying time to correct diagnosis.

Delays in treatment either due to delay in diagnosis, or secondary to fear of treatment may significantly impact outcomes. Delaying treatment can aggravate symptoms, exacerbate dysphagia and cause severe weight loss and secondary pulmonary complications such as recurrent pneumonias secondary to micro-aspirations. Untreated long-standing achalasia may result in end-stage achalasia, expressed as sigmoid esophagus on barium swallow studies and endoscopy. This entity limits the treatment options that are available for other achalasia patients who are treated earlier in the disease process. Another sequela from untreated achalasia is the increased risk for esophageal cancer. This is thought to be caused by long-standing stasis of food, liquid and debris in the esophagus resulting in bacterial overgrowth and subsequently squamous cell cancer [9].

## 2. Diagnosis and work up

The diagnosis of achalasia is determined based on findings from three studies: high-resolution esophageal manometry, contrast enhanced swallow study (CESS), and esophagogastroduodenoscopy (EGD) [10]. The clinical severity is determined based on the Eckardt score scaling system.

### 2.1 Contrast enhanced swallow study (CESS)

A key portion of diagnosis includes the evaluation of the anatomical image of the esophagus. Contrast enhanced swallow study, also known as barium swallow or upper GI swallow, allows for the visualization of the esophagus and elimination of alternative diagnosis such as carcinoma, strictures or diverticula [11]. CESS is non-invasive, widely available, and relatively inexpensive [12, 13]. As CESS has only 60% sensitivity for identifying achalasia [14], it cannot be solely relied upon for the diagnosis. The classic sign of tapering of the esophagus at the distal end giving a "bird's beak" appearance at the esophagogastric junction is pathognomonic for a diagnosis of achalasia (**Figure 1A**). Additional findings include dilation of the esophagus, retention of barium in the esophagus and an air-fluid level. In long standing disease a sigmoid shape esophagus may be evident. The absence of gastric air bubble is also suggestive of achalasia. A torturous twisting appearance of the esophagus in a "corkscrew" fashion (**Figure 1B**) may also be suggestive of esophageal dysmotility [15].

### 2.2 Esophagogastrodoudenoscopy (EGD)

EGD is important in the diagnosis of achalasia as it is necessary to rule out other possible causes of dysphagia including gastroesophageal reflux, strictures due to

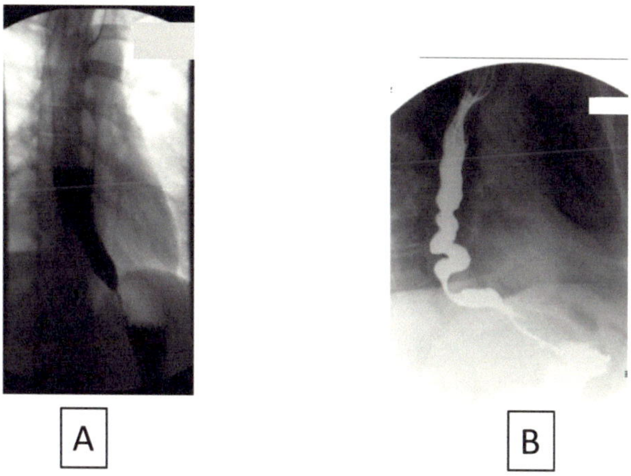


**Figure 1.**
*Contrast enhanced swallow study images that correlate with achalasia. A: Pathognomonic appearance of bird's beak on CESS. B: Corkscrew esophagus from esophageal dysmotility.*

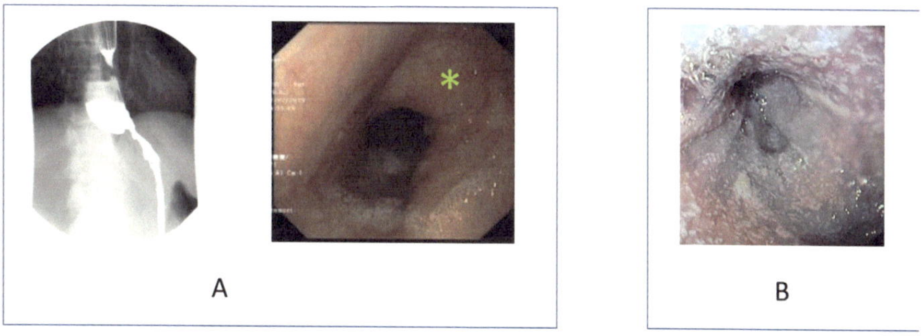


**Figure 2.**
*Endoscopic images of different endoscopic pathologies that can mimic achalasia symptoms. A: Esophageal diverticula- on the left fluoroscopic image, on the right endoscopic image (green asterisk marks the diverticula). B: Esophageal candidiasis.*

erosive esophagitis, esophageal diverticula (**Figure 2A**), tumors and obtaining biopsies to rule out eosinophilic esophagitis. Careful attention should be made to the ease of passage through the esophago-gastric junction (EGJ) into the stomach, any signs of esophagitis or strictures, as well as a detailed retroflexion view to rule out any tumor. Additional findings may include candidiasis infection (**Figure 2B**) as demonstrated by white plaques on the esophageal walls, not uncommon in patients with achalasia, most likely secondary to the change in pH due to food stasis [16].

## 2.3 High resolution manometry (HRM)

In order to understand the motility and function of the esophagus, the high-resolution manometry in conjunction with the new Chicago Classification 4.0 has allowed for better understanding, earlier diagnosis and improved classification of esophageal motility disorders [1, 17]. The HRM is able to provide images detailing the information regarding vigor of each swallow, peristalsis, relaxation and pressure of the upper and lower esophageal sphincters, thereby improving diagnostic accuracy [18]. Furthermore, the ability of testing to differentiate between the pressures of

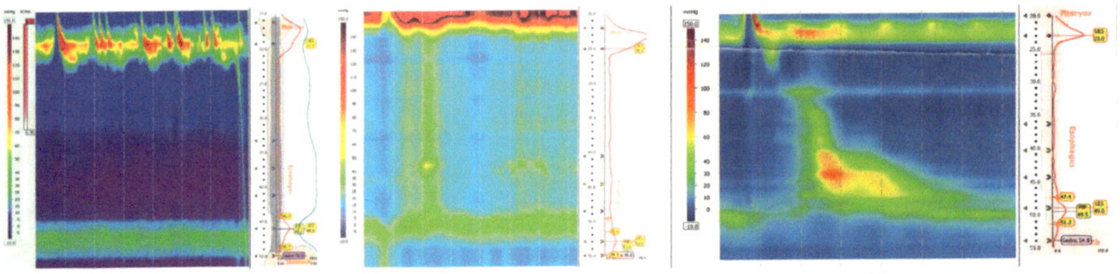


**Figure 3.**
*High resolution manometry demonstrating different types of achalasia (left to right)- all 3 types have mean IRP pressure higher than the upper limit of normal. Type 1 with 100% failed peristalsis, type 2 with panesophageal pressurization and type 3 with distal spastic contractions.*

the lower esophageal sphincter and the diaphragmatic pressure, which with previous standard manometry was not as clearly differentiated, has been beneficial. The identification of hiatal hernia versus increased esophageal pressure is one of the keys to proper diagnosis and treatment.

HRM in which a catheter containing pressure sensors approximately 1 to 2 cm apart is positioned from the hypopharynx to the stomach (via nasal introduction) with the patient being asked to swallow mouthfuls of water at several intervals. The sensors combined with computer analytic software can build an image of higher and lower pressures, peristalsis and relaxation of the esophageal sphincters. The inclusion of impedance which allows for the visualization of bolus clearance, also aides in the differentiation of esophageal from oro-pharyngeal motility dysfunctions [19].

In achalasia findings on HRM will be dependent on what type of achalasia is present, with all types demonstrating both aperistalsis and elevated Lower esophageal sphincter residual pressures (>15). Determination of which type of achalasia will be dependent on the remaining findings on HRM (**Figure 3**).

Hallmark findings according to the Chicago classification 4.0 for Type 1 achalasia will demonstrate 100% failed peristalsis, while type 2 will demonstrate panesophageal pressurization in 20% or more swallows, and type 3 will present with 20% or more premature spastic appearing contractions.

### 2.4 Eckardt score

Eckardt score (**Table 1**) is a scoring panel used to assess the severity of achalasia symptoms and is based on four major symptoms: dysphagia, regurgitation, chest pain, and weight loss [10]. Symptoms of dysphagia in patients with achalasia are usually described as progressing from solids and to liquids. Regurgitation, bringing up undigested food following meals – even hours later, is also common. Retrosternal chest pain is usually described as burning pressure often radiating to the upper back and neck. Weight loss varies, according to the dietary changes made by each patient to accommodate their symptoms.

To score, each symptom is given a value between 0 and 3 depending on its frequency (**Table 1**). It is important to note that while the Eckardt score is utilized for the determination of severity and for determining success of treatment, it holds limitations, and the severity may not correlate with manometric or CESS findings. The occurrence of concomitant obesity and achalasia has been previously reported, and as the obesity endemic grows, the possibility of achalasia in obese patients presenting with dysphagia should not be discounted [20]. As such, determination of severity based on the Eckardt scale may not accurately reflect certain populations with achalasia.

| | Weight loss (kg) | Dysphagia | Retrosternal pain | Regurgitation |
|---|---|---|---|---|
| 0 | None | None | None | None |
| 1 | <5 | Occasional | Occasional | Occasional |
| 2 | 5 to 10 | Daily | Daily | Daily |
| 3 | >10 | Each Meal | Each Meal | Each Meal |

**Table 1.**
*Eckardt score: Each symptom is given a value between 0 and 3 depending on frequency while weight loss is scored based on how many kilogram in weight have been lost. A summary of this score is done and a total between 0 and 12 is given.*

## 2.5 EndoFLIP™-

Functional luminal imaging probe (FLIP) quantifies the relationship between luminal geometry and pressure when assessing the esophageal wall and area around the lower esophageal sphincter (LES) at the esophago-gastric junction (EGJ). EndoFLIP™ (Medtronic Inc., Minneapolis, Minn, USA) provides information on both distensibility and lumen diameter of the esophagus. The technology consists of a multielectrode probe and proprietary software that measures the dynamic geometrical changes of the EGJ and esophageal body. It uses high-resolution impedance planimetry during volume-controlled distension of the probe once it passes the EGJ. Specifically, EndoFLIP analyzes the relationship between luminal cross-sectional area (CSA) and pressure, providing a measurement of the luminal distensibility (CSA/pressure) [21, 22]. The EndoFLIP can be used intraoperatively to assess treatment results following completion of myotomy (**Figure 4**). As opposed to HRM which requires patient cooperation and swallowing, the EndoFLIP can be performed on anesthetized patients and determine the post-op distensibility and lumen diameter.

In addition, there are several reports in the literature that use FLIP to evaluate contractility in the esophageal body of patients to complement HRM results. However, in

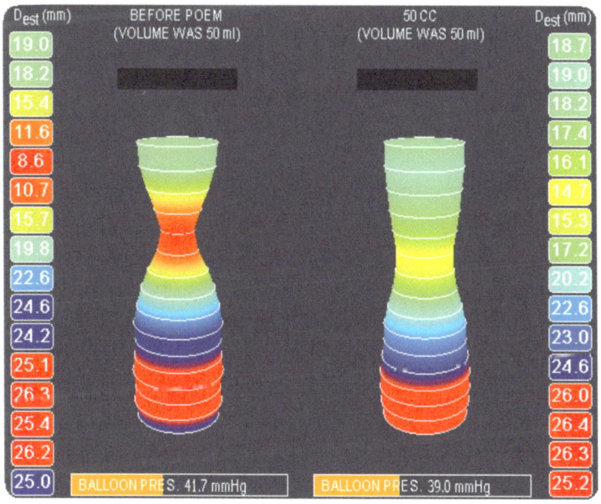


**Figure 4.**
*EndoFLIP- on the left is the pre-myotomy image showing low distensibility at the EGJ with narrow passage. On the right is the post-myotomy image showing improvement in the distensibility and a wider passage at the EGJ.*

order to do so, the probe is placed more proximal along the esophagus and a special software is used to assess peristalsis [23, 24].

## 3. Treatment options

The mainstay of treatment for achalasia is directed toward lowering the LES pressure to allow food passage to the stomach. The non-surgical treatment options include pneumatic balloon dilatation and Botulinum toxin injection while surgical treatments include Heller myotomy and per-oral endoscopic myotomy (POEM) [25, 26]. Offering the appropriate treatment option to a specific patient is done when taking into consideration all the pre-operative work up, comorbidities, and nutritional status of each individual patient.

### 3.1 Non-surgical treatment

Generally, the non-surgical treatment options are preferred for patients who are considered high risk for surgical intervention secondary to their comorbidities.

#### *3.1.1 Botiluim toxin injection*

Botilium toxin A (Allergan Inc., Irvine, California, USA), a muscle paralytic which acts via inhibiting the release of acetylcholine locally at the neuromuscular junction thereby reducing the tone of the lower esophageal sphincter resulting in its relaxation [27]. Endoscopically guided injections of 25 units are placed in each of four quadrants circumferentially around the lower esophageal sphincter just above the Z line using a sclerotherapy needle, for a total of 100 units. However, its rather limited short acting results with 78.7% patients having relief of symptoms at one month post injection and declining to 40.6% at 12 months post injection [28], and approximately 50% of patients requiring repeated injections [29]. Botilium toxin injection may be used as a bridging procedure in severely malnourished patients until surgery to allow some relief of symptoms and weight gain [30]. Botilium toxin injection may be a good option for elderly high-risk surgical patients, even if repeated injections are necessary.

#### *3.1.2 Pneumatic dilation*

Under endoscopic and radiological guidance an achalasia balloon commonly the Rigiflex Balloon system (Boston Scientific Corp, Boston, Massachusetts, USA) is used to tear the musculature of the lower esophageal sphincter thereby reducing the outflow obstruction and alleviating symptoms. The balloon should be approximately 150% of the diameter of normal EG junction. It is placed under endoscopic and fluoroscopic guidance and slowly inflated to 30 to 35 or 40 mm using 7–15 psi of air. The balloon is held inflated for 15–60 seconds effectively tearing the lower esophageal sphincter muscles thereby leaving the area open [31]. A risk of pneumatic dilation (PD) is the possibility of esophageal perforation, carrying a risk of 1.9% when done by experienced clinicians (range 0–16), and if occurs requires emergent surgical intervention. With 62% of patients reporting alleviation of symptoms at 6 months post dilation, this is a good option for poor surgical candidates [32].

It should be noted that a PD post-surgical intervention either lap heller or POEM may be useful tool for treating recurrence of symptoms (see below recurrent symptoms) [33]. Typically, a one-time treatment to 30 mm is sufficient.

## 3.2 Surgical intervention

Laparoscopic Heller myotomy (LHM) with fundoplication is the surgical gold standard treatment of achalasia. Since 2007 with the introduction of Per-Oral Endoscopic Myotomy (POEM), has become more widely used. LHM has excellent efficacy, with an improvement in symptom scores and high satisfaction in more than 90% of patients for up to 5 years after the procedure [34]. Due to the high rate of malnutrition in patients with achalasia, it is imperative to evaluate the patient's metabolic status and consider pre-operative enteral nutrition. By providing enteral or parenteral nutrition for a short time prior to surgical intervention, the catabolic status may be reversed, thereby reducing chances of complications.

### *3.2.1 Laparoscopic or robotic Heller myotomy*

Laparoscopic Heller Myotomy (LHM) includes the division of the circular and longitudinal muscles 2 cm distal and 5–7 cm proximal to the EGJ in achalasia types 1 and 2. For achalasia type 3 a longer, esophageal myotomy is done, and can be tailored to each patient according to the HRM. In order to avoid gastro- esophageal reflux, a fundoplication, either posterior (Toupet) or anterior (Dor) is added to the procedure.

This procedure can be done robotically with enhanced visualization of the circular muscles and better control of their delicate division and several studies and meta-analysis have demonstrated a lower of esophageal perforation rate and reduction of technical complications [35, 36].

Several studies have shown excellent results with LHM, demonstrating improvement of symptoms and patient satisfaction of >90% in the 6 months post-operative period. These results were maintained in most studies for up to 5 years. However, there were some studies demonstrating a decrease with time in symptoms improvement of up to 57% in some reports [32, 34, 37]. Although LHM is done with fundoplication, some patients still suffer from GERD symptoms and have esophagitis on endoscopy.

### *3.2.2 Per-Oral endoscopic myotomy (POEM)*

Once considered innovative novel procedure, POEM is becoming more and more accepted as a viable alternative to LHM. POEM is performed under general anesthesia using a standard gastroscope inserted into the esophagus per orally.

A small longitudinal incision is made on the esophageal mucosa approximately 10 cm proximal to the EGJ to allow the gastroscope to slide into the submucosal plane. A sub-mucosal dissection is then performed and carried all the way until 2 cm distal to the EGJ. Then the myotomy is performed including the circular muscle layer only, leaving the longitudinal layer intact. The length of the myotomy is tailored to each patient according to the HRM but usually begins from 2 cm distal to the EGJ to 5–7 cm proximal to it. This can be done in an antegrade fashion or retrograde. It can be done on the anterior or the posterior aspects of the esophagus [38]. POEM is especially recommended for patients with type 3 achalasia as a long thoracic myotomy is indicated for these patients [39], which is more difficult to perform in LHM.

POEM has excellent results as demonstrated by a reduction in Eckardt score to <3, achieving clinical success and improvement of dysphagia in 83–98% of the patients [40, 41]. However, GERD is a concern among post-operative achalasia patients. Several studies have compared LHM to POEM regarding post-operative GERD symptoms. Werner et al. [41] randomly assigned 221 patients to undergo either POEM (112 patients) or LHM plus Dor's fundoplication (109 patients). They showed that after POEM 44% of the patients had esophagitis after 24 months vs. 29% in the LHM group. However, high-grade esophagitis (Los Angeles Classification grade C or D) was similar between POEM and LHM at 24 months, suggesting 5% in the POEM group and 6% in the LHM group. They also found that 24 h pH monitoring was similar among patients who underwent POEM and LHM.

In order to reduce reflux symptoms that could potentially lead to GERD, esophagitis, strictures, Barrett's esophagus and even cancer Inoue et al. [42] described adding an endoscopic fundoplication to POEM (F-POEM), but this technique is still novel and needs to be further explored.

#### *3.2.3 Esophagectomy*

End-stage achalasia is characterized by severe dysphagia and a sigmoid, torturous esophagus seen on endoscopy and on barium swallow study. Although patients with end-stage achalasia might suffer from complications such as pulmonary complications, esophagitis and risk for cancer, they do not have many treatment options [43]. Although most studies suggest that POEM, LHM or PD might be the first step in trying to treat patients with end-stage achalasia [44, 45], others suggest that esophagectomy alone is the treatment that these patients should be offered [46].

Reconstruction after esophagectomy can be done preferably using gastric pull-up or colonic interposition. This is a high morbidity procedure that should be reserved to specific patients as it comes with the potential for significant post-operative complications, morbidity and although rare, mortality [47, 48].

## 4. Special considerations

### 4.1 Pediatric population

In recent years, the incidence of achalasia has risen rather significantly including an increase in pediatric population and may in part be due to the increased sensitivity of testing and increased awareness of the diagnosis. Children who were otherwise misdiagnosed, with anorexia, chronic pulmonary manifestations such as recurrent pneumonia and failure to thrive are now being diagnosed with achalasia. Diagnosis is made as in the adult population, via HRM, EGD and CESS. Special attention should be made to biopsies for evaluation of eosinophilic esophagitis which may mimic achalasia symptoms but requires treatment with oral steroid gel rather than surgical intervention. In general, the treatment options for the pediatric population need to take into consideration growth and long-term risk for reflux. The gold standard of treatment in pediatric patients is laparoscopic Heller myotomy Botilium toxin injection is not recommended as there is no clear dose known for pediatric population [49]. Pneumatic dilation is not a good option for children as first line therapy, due to need for recurrent dilations [50]. In recent years, POEM has gained popularity and is often preferred over traditional surgery. With results similar to their adult counterparts, POEM is a good option for pediatric population in the hands of experienced surgeons [51, 52].

### 4.2 Pregnancy

Maternal nutrition has long been a subject in the medical world and similar to malnutrition from other causes, achalasia is known to cause intrauterine growth restriction, preterm labor and small for gestational age [53]. Additional considerations include the socioeconomic effects of absent mothers due to extended hospitalizations, missed work, and increased healthcare costs. The early diagnosis and treatment of achalasia prior to pregnancy is imperative to ensure healthy outcomes for both mother and fetus. As such ideally, diagnosis and treatment are made prior to pregnancy. However, in cases where the diagnosis is only made during pregnancy the clinician must take into consideration both patients, mother and fetus. Treatment options during pregnancy may include enteral nutrition supplements via feeding tube placement and delaying definitive treatment until delivery with close monitoring of fetus for IUGR and SGA.

Non-surgical treatments such as Botox injection have been reported in the literature [54, 55] however, Botox is labeled as a pregnancy category C, based on studies using significantly lower doses for cosmetic use. As such the use Botox in pregnancy and its safety is not clear [56].

Following delivery, standard surgical intervention can be scheduled either laparoscopic Heller myotomy or POEM.

### 4.3 Follow up

Post POEM follow up should include surveillance with Eckardt score, with a score less than three regarded as treatment success, barium swallow study, 24 hours pH-metry, manometry and EGD as needed based on patient symptomatology [57]. While follow up diagnostics and treatments vary from center to center, studies have found that surveillance EGD at 1 year post POEM may help to identify those patients with reflux [58]. The recommendation for yearly EGD examination has also been suggested by Milito et al. [59].

### 4.4 Salvage therapy for recurrence or failed treatment

Recurrence of symptoms can occur in some patients. These symptoms need to be investigated to understand if the symptoms are related to outflow obstruction, GERD or dysmotility of the esophagus. A barium swallow study should be performed for an accurate imaging of the esophagus with dynamic evaluation, an upper endoscopy to assess the LES, presence of esophagitis, candidiasis or other pathology and a manometry to evaluate the esophagus and the LES function. If available, EndoFLIP is a reasonable complementary test for evaluation.

After these assessments, if a diagnosis of recurrence or failed treatment is established, a salvage therapy may be offered. The salvage therapy depends on the type of initial treatment. Studies trying to evaluate what kind of salvage therapy is more appropriate, failed to demonstrated superiority of one over the other [60–63]. After failed LHM or POEM either posterior POEM or PD can be offered. If a patient suffers from GERD after POEM a treatment with either medical management or laparoscopic fundoplication are viable options. In patients with candida which can mimic recurrence of symptoms, the recommended treatment is oral antifungals.

## 5. Summary

While achalasia was once thought to be a rare disorder, recent years has seen a significant increase in the incidence, perhaps attributable to the increased use of HRM and general recognition of the disease. Contrary to classic textbook descriptions, achalasia patients may present in normal weight or even obese due to the availability of high calorie and protein soft and liquid food. Diagnosis should be made based on three exams, HRM, CESS and EGD. The Eckardt score can aid in understanding the severity of symptoms, but may not adequately reflect actual disease status, and may not be correlated with exam findings. Early treatment is key especially in younger populations, in order to prevent disease progression and complications. Treatment options should be tailored to each patient based on age, nutrition status and comorbidities. The gold standard of treatment is Laparoscopic Heller Myotomy with fundoplication; however, POEM has been accepted as a comparable surgical treatment if performed in experienced centers. Follow-up is mandatory to assist patients with coping with this chronic disease and screen for early or late complications as well as offering salvage treatment when needed.

Achalasia is a chronic and irreversible condition. Early treatment may slow down the progression of the disease. Opening the LES may facilitate passage of food into the stomach and alleviate symptoms, however aperistalsis of the esophagus persists.

## Author details

Gad Marom[1,2]*, Ronit Brodie[1] and Yoav Mintz[1,2]

1 Department of General Surgery, Hadassah Hebrew University Medical Center, Jerusalem, Israel

2 Faculty of Medicine, Hebrew University of Jerusalem, Jerusalem, Israel

*Address all correspondence to: gadimarom@gmail.com

## References

[1] Yadlapati R et al. Esophageal motility disorders on high-resolution manometry: Chicago classification version 4.0(©). Neurogastroenterology and Motility. 2021;**33**(1):e14058

[2] Eckardt VF, Aignherr C, Bernhard G. Predictors of outcome in patients with achalasia treated by pneumatic dilation. Gastroenterology. 1992;**103**(6):1732-1738

[3] Samo S et al. Incidence and prevalence of achalasia in Central Chicago, 2004-2014, since the widespread use of high-resolution manometry. Clinical Gastroenterology and Hepatology. 2017;**15**(3):366-373

[4] Duffield JA et al. Incidence of achalasia in South Australia based on esophageal manometry findings. Clinical Gastroenterology and Hepatology. 2017;**15**(3):360-365

[5] Annese V, Bassotti G. Non-surgical treatment of esophageal achalasia. World Journal of Gastroenterology. 2006;**12**(36):5763-5766

[6] Howard PJ et al. Five year prospective study of the incidence, clinical features, and diagnosis of achalasia in Edinburgh. Gut. 1992;**33**(8):1011-1015

[7] Goldacre M, Benians R, Goldacre R. Esophageal achalasia diagnosed in people previously diagnosed with an eating disorder: Epidemiological study using record-linkage. The International Journal of Eating Disorders. 2021;**54**(11): 2015-2018

[8] Letranchant A et al. Eating disorder or oesophageal achalasia during adolescence: Diagnostic difficulties. Eating and Weight Disorders. 2020;**25**(1): 87-90

[9] Chino O et al. Clinicopathological studies of esophageal carcinoma in achalasia: Analyses of carcinogenesis using histological and immunohistochemical procedures. Anticancer Research. 2000;**20**(5c):3717-3722

[10] Eckardt AJ, Eckardt VF. Current clinical approach to achalasia. World Journal of Gastroenterology. 2009;**15**(32):3969-3975

[11] Schlottmann F, Patti MG. Esophageal achalasia: Current diagnosis and treatment. Expert Review of Gastroenterology & Hepatology. 2018;**12**(7):711-721

[12] Aviv JE et al. Cost-effectiveness of two types of dysphagia care in head and neck cancer: A preliminary report. Ear, Nose, & Throat Journal. 2001;**80**(8):553-556 558

[13] Administration HCF. Enrollment Package, Medicare Part B, Area 01, Manhattan. Washington DC: H.C.F. Administration; 2000

[14] El-Takli I, O'Brien P, Paterson WG. Clinical diagnosis of achalasia: How reliable is the barium x-ray? Canadian Journal of Gastroenterology. 2006;**20**(5):335-337

[15] Debi U et al. Barium esophagogram in various esophageal diseases: A pictorial essay. Indian Journal of Radiology and Imaging. 2019;**29**(2):141-154

[16] Pandolfino JE, Gawron AJ. Achalasia: A systematic review. JAMA. 2015;**313**(18):1841-1852

[17] Lafraia FM et al. A pictorial presentation of esophageal high

resolution manometry current parameters. Arquivos Brasileiros de Cirurgia Digestiva. 2017;**30**(1):69-71

[18] Pandolfino JE et al. High-resolution manometry in clinical practice: Utilizing pressure topography to classify oesophageal motility abnormalities. Neurogastroenterology and Motility. 2009;**21**(8):796-806

[19] Carlson DA, Pandolfino JE. High-resolution manometry in clinical practice. Gastroenterology & Hepatology (N Y). 2015;**11**(6):374-384

[20] Almogy G, Anthone GJ, Crookes PF. Achalasia in the context of morbid obesity: A rare but important association. Obesity Surgery. 2003;**13**(6):896-900

[21] Savarino E et al. Use of the functional lumen imaging probe in clinical Esophagology. The American Journal of Gastroenterology. 2020;**115**(11):1786-1796

[22] Pannala R et al. Devices for esophageal function testing. VideoGIE. 2022;**7**(1):1-20

[23] Carlson DA et al. Classifying esophageal motility by FLIP Panometry: A study of 722 subjects with manometry. The American Journal of Gastroenterology. 2021;**116**(12):2357-2366

[24] Carlson DA et al. The functional lumen imaging probe detects esophageal contractility not observed with manometry in patients with achalasia. Gastroenterology. 2015;**149**(7):1742-1751

[25] Khashab MA et al. ASGE guideline on the management of achalasia. Gastrointestinal Endoscopy. 2020;**91**(2):213-227.e6

[26] Tolone S et al. Recent trends in endoscopic management of achalasia. World Journal of Gastrointestinal Endoscopy. 2014;**6**(9):407-414

[27] Brisinda G et al. Treatment of gastrointestinal sphincters spasms with botulinum toxin a. Toxins (Basel). 2015;**7**(6):1882-1916

[28] Campos GM et al. Endoscopic and surgical treatments for achalasia: A systematic review and meta-analysis. Annals of Surgery. 2009;**249**(1):45-57

[29] Pasricha PJ et al. Intrasphincteric botulinum toxin for the treatment of achalasia. The New England Journal of Medicine. 1995;**332**(12):774-778

[30] DeMeester SR. Per-oral endoscopic myotomy for achalasia. Journal of Thoracic Disease. 2017;**9**(Suppl. 2): S130-s134

[31] Richter JE. Esophageal motility disorder achalasia. Current Opinion in Otolaryngology & Head and Neck Surgery. 2013;**21**(6):535-542

[32] Vela MF et al. The long-term efficacy of pneumatic dilatation and Heller myotomy for the treatment of achalasia. Clinical Gastroenterology and Hepatology. 2006;**4**(5):580-587

[33] Patti MG, Schlottmann F, Herbella FAM. Esophageal achalasia: Evaluation and treatment of recurrent symptoms. World Journal of Surgery. 2022;**46**(7):1561-1566

[34] Ortiz A et al. Very long-term objective evaluation of heller myotomy plus posterior partial fundoplication in patients with achalasia of the cardia. Annals of Surgery. 2008;**247**(2):258-264

[35] Milone M et al. Robotic versus laparoscopic approach to treat symptomatic achalasia: Systematic

review with meta-analysis. Diseases of the Esophagus. 2019;**32**(10):1-8

[36] Ali AB et al. Robotic and per-oral endoscopic myotomy have fewer technical complications compared to laparoscopic Heller myotomy. Surgical Endoscopy. 2020;**34**(7):3191-3196

[37] Patti MG, Tamburini A, Pellegrini CA. Cardiomyotomy. Seminars in Laparoscopic Surgery. 1999;**6**(4): 186-193

[38] Marom G et al. The POEM bottom-up technique for achalasia. Surgical Endoscopy. 2021;**35**(11):6117-6122

[39] Vaezi MF et al. ACG clinical guidelines: Diagnosis and Management of Achalasia. The American Journal of Gastroenterology. 2020;**115**(9):1393-1411

[40] Delliturri A et al. A narrative review of update in per oral endoscopic myotomy (POEM) and endoscopic esophageal surgery. Annals of Translational Medicine. 2021;**9**(10):909

[41] Werner YB et al. Endoscopic or surgical Myotomy in patients with idiopathic achalasia. The New England Journal of Medicine. 2019;**381**(23):2219-2229

[42] Inoue H et al. Peroral endoscopic myotomy and fundoplication: A novel NOTES procedure. Endoscopy. 2019;**51**(2):161-164

[43] Eckardt VF, Hoischen T, Bernhard G. Life expectancy, complications, and causes of death in patients with achalasia: Results of a 33-year follow-up investigation. European Journal of Gastroenterology & Hepatology. 2008;**20**(10):956-960

[44] Qiu S et al. Advanced achalasia: Good candidate for peroral endoscopic myotomy. Diseases of the Esophagus. 2021;**34**(3):1-7

[45] Waters J, Martin LW, Molena D. Esophagectomy for end-stage achalasia. World Journal of Surgery. 2022;**46**(7): 1567-1574

[46] Devaney EJ et al. Esophagectomy for achalasia: Patient selection and clinical experience. The Annals of Thoracic Surgery. 2001;**72**(3):854-858

[47] Glatz SM, Richardson JD. Esophagectomy for end stage achalasia. Journal of Gastrointestinal Surgery. 2007;**11**(9):1134-1137

[48] Palanivelu C et al. Laparoscopic transhiatal esophagectomy for 'sigmoid' megaesophagus following failed cardiomyotomy: Experience of 11 patients. Digestive Diseases and Sciences. 2008;**53**(6):1513-1518

[49] Franklin AL, Petrosyan M, Kane TD. Childhood achalasia: A comprehensive review of disease, diagnosis and therapeutic management. World Journal of Gastrointestinal Endoscopy. 2014;**6**(4):105-111

[50] Tashiro J, Petrosyan M, Kane TD. Current management of pediatric achalasia. Translational Gastroenterology and Hepatology. 2021;**6**:33

[51] Goneidy A et al. Surgical Management of Esophageal Achalasia in pediatrics: A systematic review. European Journal of Pediatric Surgery. 2020;**30**(1):13-20

[52] Choné A et al. Multicenter evaluation of clinical efficacy and safety of per-oral endoscopic Myotomy in children. Journal of Pediatric Gastroenterology and Nutrition. 2019;**69**(5):523-527

[53] Khudyak V, Lysy J, Mankuta D. Achalasia in pregnancy. Obstetrical &

Gynecological Survey. 2006;**61**(3): 207-211

[54] Hooft N, Schmidt ES, Bremner RM. Achalasia in pregnancy: Botulinum toxin a injection of lower esophageal sphincter. Case Reports Surgery. 2015;**2015**:328970

[55] Wataganara T et al. Treatment of severe achalasia during pregnancy with esophagoscopic injection of botulinum toxin a: A case report. Journal of Perinatology. 2009;**29**(9):637-639

[56] Lowe NJ et al. Dosing, efficacy and safety plus the use of computerized photography for botulinum toxins type a for upper facial lines. Journal of Cosmetic and Laser Therapy. 2010;**12**(2):106-111

[57] Oude Nijhuis RAB et al. European guidelines on achalasia: United European gastroenterology and European Society of Neurogastroenterology and Motility recommendations. United European. Gastroenterologisches Journal. 2020;**8**(1):13-33

[58] Ponds FA et al. Effect of Peroral endoscopic Myotomy vs pneumatic dilation on symptom severity and treatment outcomes among treatment-naive patients with achalasia: A randomized clinical trial. JAMA. 2019;**322**(2):134-144

[59] Milito P et al. Revisional therapy for recurrent symptoms after Heller Myotomy for achalasia. Journal of Gastrointestinal Surgery. 2022;**26**(1):64-69

[60] Felix VN et al. Achalasia: What to do in the face of failures of Heller myotomy. Annals of the New York Academy of Sciences. 2020;**1481**(1):236-246

[61] Legros L et al. Long-term results of pneumatic dilatation for relapsing symptoms of achalasia after Heller myotomy. Neurogastroenterology and Motility. 2014;**26**(9):1248-1255

[62] Tang X et al. Feasibility and safety of peroral endoscopic myotomy for achalasia after failed endoscopic interventions. Diseases of the Esophagus. 2017;**30**(3):1-6

[63] van Hoeij FB et al. Management of recurrent symptoms after per-oral endoscopic myotomy in achalasia. Gastrointestinal Endoscopy. 2018;**87**(1):95-101

Chapter 5

# Gastric Volvulus

*Maria Carolina Jimenez, Jose M. Martinez and Robert F. Cubas*

## Abstract

Gastric volvulus is one of the most worrisome complications related to large paraesophageal hernias. It is a medical emergency that requires high index of suspicion and prompt management and operation during the index admission. Here we discuss the pathophysiology and classification of gastric volvulus, clinical and radiological presentation, and treatment options. The approaches described here include endoscopic, laparoscopic, robotic and open. We advocate for the first three approaches and usually save the open approach for certain redo operations or patients with significant adhesions from prior mediastinal or foregut surgeries.

**Keywords:** gastric volvulus, paraesophageal hernia, gastropexy, endoscopy, hernia

## 1. Introduction

Gastric volvulus, from the Latin volvere (meaning 'to roll'), is an uncommon clinical entity, occurring in both adult and pediatric populations and defined as the pathological rotation of the stomach beyond 180 degrees. It was first described by Berti in 1866 based on the autopsy of a woman who died of closed loop obstruction and Berg described the first operation in 1897. It is considered a life-threatening emergency due to formation of a closed loop obstruction with strangulation which can progress to gastric ischemia, necrosis and perforation [1–9].

Its true incidence is unknown because besides being a rare condition, many chronic cases are never diagnosed. The clinical presentation is variable and may range from an intermittent non-specific abdominal pain to acute abdomen requiring emergency surgery. The mortality rate for acute volvulus ranges from 30–50%, highlighting the importance of early diagnosis and treatment [2, 3, 5, 10].

## 2. Pathophysiology

Primary gastric volvulus refers to the absence of diaphragmatic defects or intra-abdominal abnormality causing the volvulus, accounting for approximately 30% of cases [2, 6, 10]. The stomach is fixed to the abdominal wall by the gastrocolic, gastrohepatic, gastrophrenic, and gastrosplenic ligaments. Together with the gastroesophageal junction and the pylorus, these ligaments provide anchorage and prevent malrotation. When these mechanisms fail, the patient may be at risk of primary gastric volvulus [5, 6].

Secondary gastric volvulus may arise due to disorders of gastric anatomy or gastric function or abnormalities of adjacent organs such as the diaphragm or spleen. Up to 75% are associated with a paraesophageal hernia (PEH), diaphragmatic hernia, wandering spleen, abdominal adhesions, diaphragmatic eventration, phrenic nerve paralysis, or other diaphragmatic or intraabdominal conditions [1–3, 5, 6, 10, 11].

Risk factors include age over 50, gastric ligament laxity, pyloric stenosis, gastroduodenal tumors, diaphragmatic injury and eventration, left lung resection, or pleural adhesions [2].

The fifth decade is the age group with the highest incidence with children less than one year old making up 10–20% of cases. No association with either sex or race has been reported [2, 3, 5, 6, 10].

## 3. Classification

Several anatomopathological classifications have been proposed, and the most complete one was proposed by Von Haberer and Singleton, modified by Carter in 1978 describing three types of gastric volvulus according to the axis of rotation: organoaxial, mesenteroaxial and combined [1, 2, 5, 11].

Organoaxial volvulus is a rotation of the stomach around a longitudinal axis passing through the cardia and the pylorus. It is the most common form, occurring in approximately 60% of cases. The most common causes of this subtype are paraesophageal hernias and diaphragmatic eventration. It causes the greater curvature of the stomach to rest superior to the lesser curvature, resulting in an 'inverted' stomach. The distinguishing feature of this variant is that it lies in the horizontal plane when viewed on plain radiography **Figure 1** [1, 2, 5, 11].

The second type of gastric volvulus is mesenteroaxial. It is a less common subtype, comprising approximately 29% of cases. Rotation occurs along a transverse axis, passing through the midpoints of the small and the great curvature. This type is more likely found in the pediatric population and is rarely described in adult individuals. Strangulation is less likely to occur due to spontaneous detorsions with recurrent acute episodes **Figure 2** [1, 2, 5, 11].

The third and rarest subtype of gastric volvulus is when the stomach rotates about both the organo-axial and mesenteroaxial axes resulting in a combined volvulus [1, 2, 5, 11].

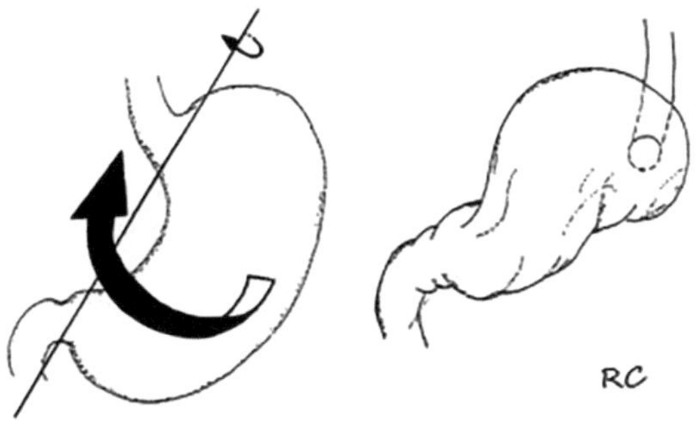


**Figure 1.**
*Organoaxial volvulus.*

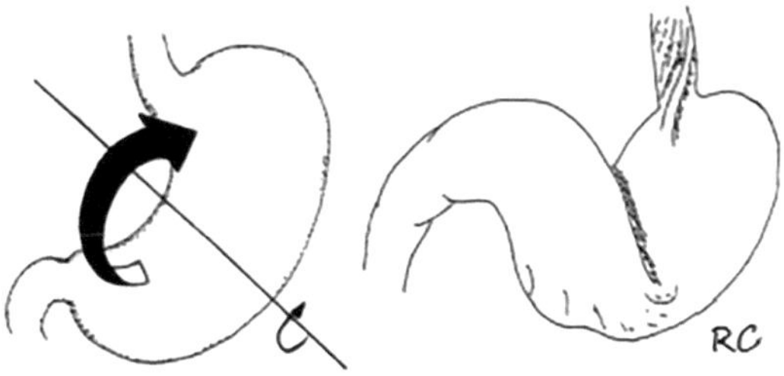


**Figure 2.**
*Mesenteroaxial volvulus.*

## 4. Clinical presentation

The clinical presentation of patients with gastric volvulus depends on the speed of onset, type of volvulus and degree of obstruction [1, 5].

Given that gastric volvulus is a rare condition, it is rarely considered at the top of the differential diagnoses when a patient presents with abdominal, or chest pain associated with nausea and vomiting [5].

The classic symptoms, known as "Borchardt's triad," consist of:

- Nonproductive vomiting
- Epigastric pain, and
- Difficulty inserting a nasogastric (NG) tube

However, these symptoms may not be present in as many as 25% of patients. Hematemesis may also be seen and is thought to occur due to mucosal sloughing as a result of ischemia or a mucosal tear due to retching [1, 2, 4–6, 10].

On physical exam there are a variety of possible characteristic findings such as gastric sounds audible in the chest, abdominal distention and dullness to percussion. Once the disease has progressed to peritonitis, abdominal wall rigidity and rebound tenderness may also be found [6].

In contrast, chronic or intermittent gastric volvulus may present with nonspecific symptoms which may go unnoticed. These include mild upper abdominal pain, chest pain, dysphagia, bloating, early satiety, heartburn, and occasionally symptoms of pancreatitis. Such features may be protracted and are often misattributed to other upper gastrointestinal disorders such as peptic ulcer disease [4–6, 11].

Laboratory findings include [6]:

- Elevated markers of inflammation (e.g., white cell count, c-reactive protein)
- Electrolyte abnormalities (e.g., hypokalemia, hypochloremic metabolic alkalosis)
- Elevated pancreatic enzymes; and
- Anemia (related to mucosal ulceration)

Reported complications of gastric volvulus include ulceration, perforation, hemorrhage, pancreatic necrosis, and omental avulsion. On rare occasions, rotation of the stomach may even cause disruption of the splenic vessels resulting in hemorrhage and splenic rupture [5, 12].

## 5. Diagnosis

Diagnosis based on physical examination findings and symptoms alone is difficult, therefore a high index of suspicion is required, as it is a condition with a high mortality rate in acute cases [3, 4].

The gold standard is a barium swallow, which has a very high sensitivity and specificity for diagnosing gastric volvulus [10]. However, the increased availability of computed tomography has displaced barium swallow to a second place in the diagnostic armamentarium.

The diagnosis is frequently made by an abdominal radiograph and an upper gastrointestinal series, although the results may be normal during the asymptomatic period [2, 4, 11, 13].

In a typical presentation of gastric volvulus, an erect abdominal radiograph may demonstrate double air-fluid levels in the antrum and fundus, a single air bubble with no additional luminal gas or a distended fluid-filled stomach. Chest radiographs also can demonstrate a retrocardiac, air-filled mass. These features may be absent in cases of intermittent obstruction and therefore further imaging is often necessary to confirm diagnosis [5].

Upper gastrointestinal series can provide information on the rotation of the stomach and passage of ingested oral contrast material into the duodenum [4]. However, it is usually not performed routinely in mild cases due to the vagueness of symptoms and low suspicion of gastric volvulus.

Most patients, particularly those with acute abdominal pain, undergo CT scan. CT of the abdomen or chest typically demonstrates a dilated stomach, often abnormally positioned in the chest. A swirl sign may also be evident. CT also defines other anatomic abnormalities, such as diaphragmatic defects, and excludes other abdominal pathology as the source of symptoms [6]. The most frequent and sensitive CT findings of volvulus are stenosis at the hernia neck and transition point at the pylorus [4]. CT findings of ischemia including gastric wall edema, lack of contrast enhancement of the gastric wall, perigastric fluid, pneumatosis of the gastric wall, pleural effusion, and pneumoperitoneum could also be seen [2, 4, 11, 13].

Gastric volvulus can sometimes be initially diagnosed through upper endoscopy where tortuous appearance of the stomach and difficulty or inability for the endoscope to reach the pylorus may be found [2, 11]. It is also typical to see the pylorus adjacent to the esophagogastric junction on retroflexion.

## 6. Treatment

The treatment of acute gastric volvulus is medical, endoscopic and/or surgical.

### 6.1 Initial management

Initial treatment involves stabilization of the patient, balanced crystalloid resuscitation, correction of electrolyte abnormalities and urgent upper endoscopy with placement of NG tube for decompression, which will assist with reduction of the gastric volvulus and evaluation of the mucosa [6, 11, 14]. Blood-based resuscitation should be considered for patients with chronic anemia from this condition or presenting with acute upper gastrointestinal bleed. In the presence of suspected perforation or ischemia, broad spectrum antibiotics should be administered early [14].

Some authors consider that chronic gastric volvulus can be managed conservatively with prokinetic agents and antisecretory therapy [2].

Immediate surgical consultation should be obtained, particularly in the case of an acute volvulus where the risk of vascular compromise and death are high [5].

Urgent surgery is mandated in the following instances [6]:

- Inability to decompress the stomach with a nasogastric tube or endoscopy
- Gastric perforation
- Mediastinal collection
- Shock or hypotension refractory to resuscitation
- Severe sepsis

### 6.2 Endoscopy

An upper endoscopy may be initially attempted to manually reduce the hernia in stable patients, particularly when unable to pass an NG tube. If successful, this will allow further assessment of the extent of damage as a result of the volvulus and will allow time to resuscitate the patient prior to surgery. Many times decompression of the stomach with a nasogastric tube will result in reduction of the volvulus [3, 14].

The airway should be secured prior to endoscopic intervention to avoid aspiration during the procedure. Once the endoscope is inserted, esophageal and gastric contents can be suctioned and NG or orogastric tube can be guided under endoscopic visualization into the stomach for decompression [14].

Endoscopic derotation with endoscopic gastropexy via percutaneous endoscopic gastrostomy (PEG) tube has been described as conservative first-line management in patients with isolated gastric volvulus and high surgical risk [5, 10, 11, 14]. The rationale for placement of a PEG tube is that it helps prevent recurrent volvulus by fixing the stomach to the abdominal wall in its normal orientation. In the rare case that PEG is used as the sole therapy, a second PEG tube will be needed to prevent future rotation. In such cases, one PEG is placed in the usual position in the gastric body while the other is placed more distal in the stomach [14].

However, the risk of gastric perforation with endoscopic therapy as main treatment is significant and patients should therefore be considered carefully for conservative treatment [2, 10]. There is also a risk of recurrence due to inadequate fixation, persistence of predisposing factors such as hernias and adhesions from previous surgeries, and the potential that the fixation point will act as an axis for further rotations **Figure 3** [11].

### 6.3 Surgery

Surgical management is aimed at ensuring gastric viability [15]. The principles of treatment of gastric volvulus include decompression of the stomach with reduction

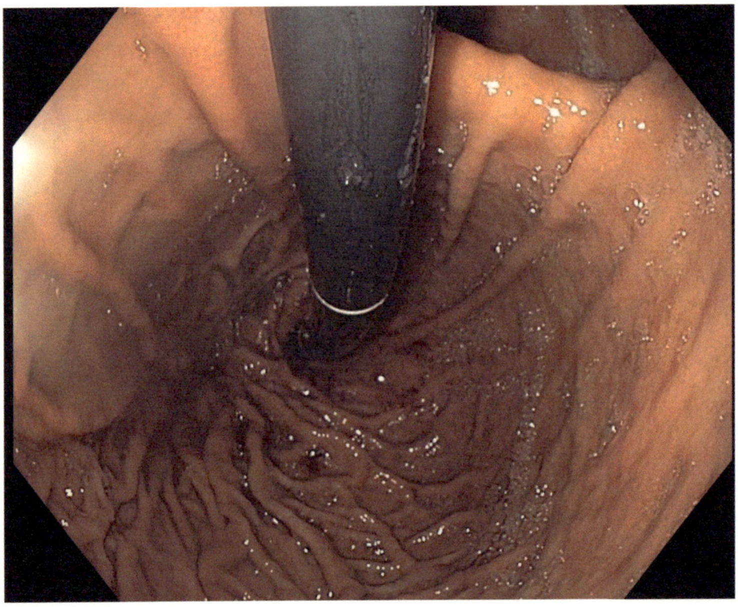

**Figure 3.**
*Endoscopic view of devolvulized stomach.*

of the volvulus to restore the stomach to a more normal anatomic position, followed by gastropexy and correction of the intra-abdominal factors predisposing to volvulus and thus preventing future stomach rotation. Gastric resection is necessary if full-thickness necrosis is present [5–7, 11, 16].

Traditionally, open surgery has been the preferred approach, allowing broad access to the abdominal cavity [1, 2, 6, 17]. Patients demonstrating signs of metabolic derangement or necrosis might benefit from open transabdominal damage-control laparotomy for reduction and relief of ischemia or resection of necrotic tissue and planned second look for definitive repair [14].

Due to the paucity of literature comparing laparoscopic and open surgery it is difficult to compare their respective outcomes. However, laparoscopic surgery has largely demonstrated its usefulness in elective surgery for chronic gastric volvulus and increasingly in cases of acute volvulus [7, 11, 12, 16–18]. Koger and Stone in 1993 described the first successful laparoscopic treatment of acute gastric volvulus by performing reduction and gastropexy [11]. Over time, good results with laparoscopic approaches have been described for gastric volvulus in stable patients, but its use in cases of perforation remains controversial [19].

Channer et al. have reported successful reduction of organoaxial gastric volvulus using standard laparoscopic foregut port placement in a small series [12]. Yates et al. have modified the port configuration to allow for sutured gastropexy of the distal gastric body and antrum [18].

In high-operative risk patients, management of gastric volvulus with laparoscopic paraesophageal hernia (PEH) repair can result in significant perioperative morbidity and mortality, and in the presence of severe thoracoabdominal musculoskeletal deformities the repair may turn into a technically challenging one [18].

Laparoscopic gastropexy requires much shorter operative time compared with laparoscopic PEH repair, possibly resulting in less perioperative morbidity and mortality for patients [8, 18]. Many technical variations of gastropexy have been reported in the literature and include [1, 5, 12, 17]:

- Simple fixation of stomach to the anterior abdominal wall, including using T-fasteners (Ross Products Division, Abbott Laboratories, Columbus, Ohio) [12] and intracorporeal suturing

- Gastrostomy tube placement

- Suturing the lesser curvature to ligamentum teres or a free edge of liver

- Posterior fixation of the greater curvature to the peritoneum and colonic mesentery

- Fixation of the fundus to the undersurface of the diaphragm

In the past, more definitive procedures that were performed included gastropexy with colonic displacement (Tanner's procedure), fundoantral gastrostomy (Oozler's operation), gastrojejunostomy and gastrocolic disconnection. However, these are rarely used nowadays.

Laparoscopic approach with excision of the hernia sac, re-approximation of the diaphragmatic crura, anti-reflux procedure and gastropexy, when indicated, has been tolerated, securing the stomach intra-abdominally and preventing migration of the stomach to an intrathoracic position. Complete excision of the hernia sac can also help to eliminate one of the causes of recurrence [12].

Due to the robust collateral circulation of the stomach, gastric necrosis is unusual, but the stomach should always be thoroughly examined for evidence of ischemia after reduction of the gastric volvulus. When it occurs, gastric necrosis is usually located at the fundus, which is a location amenable to partial resection with a linear stapler [6]. It is crucial to perform an intraoperative upper endoscopy to be able to evaluate the condition of the mucosa and the repair performed.

In the rare case of full thickness necrosis of the stomach with absence of perfusion after reduction of volvulus, a total gastrectomy may be required, leaving the esophagus and duodenum in discontinuity, placing a feeding jejunostomy tube and creating a diverting esophagostomy at the initial surgery for damage control. Once the patient is more stable, they can be taken back for definitive repair with esophagojejunal reconstruction or colonic interposition [6].

While there has been debate in the literature concerning the indications of an additional anti-reflux procedure when repairing a diaphragmatic defect, Fundoplication, especially if the wrap is sutured to the crura, has shown to decrease recurrence in patients with hiatal hernia [2, 10]. An anti-reflux procedure should be performed routinely in patients with PEH [12, 20].

More recently robotic-assisted surgery has been gaining popularity in General Surgery, and there are increasing reports demonstrating that robotic approach to the management of GERD and PEH repair is safe and effective with low complication rates [21, 22]. To date, there are very few case reports of robotic repair

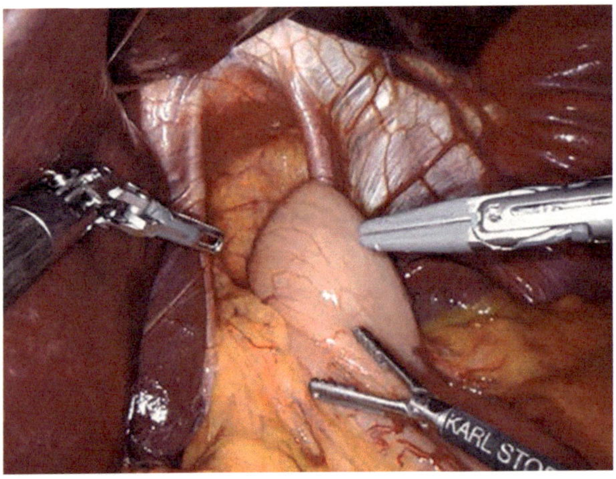


**Figure 4.**
*Robotic repair of paraesophageal hernia presenting with a gastric volvulus.*

of paraesophageal hernia with finding of gastric volvulus in children and adults **Figure 4** [21, 23–25].

### 6.4 Postoperative considerations

Postoperatively, patients should be admitted to an appropriate level of care based on clinical condition. Antiemetics should be scheduled to help prevent retching and vomiting. Currently there are no guidelines on postoperative use of NG tube or timing of enteral feeding.

Some authors tend to leave an NGT in situ, while others do not routinely leave one. Some surgeons perform a barium swallow within the first 2 postoperative days to interrogate the hernia repair, assess gastric emptying and evaluate for the presence of an esophageal leak [7, 14, 15]. We do not routinely follow this approach at our institution, unless there has been transmural gastric violation requiring repair or partial gastrectomy.

There is variety in practice with respect to feeding after surgery. We sequentially advance diet (full liquids, puree or blended diet and soft diet) for a period of 6 weeks to allow the edema at the site of the operation to resolve. Other surgeons discharge patients on a soft diet for 2 to 3 weeks after emergency repair of gastric volvulus [7, 15].

When placing a gastrostomy tube, Yates et al. typically leave it connected to a gravity bag for 12 to 24 hours postoperatively. Thereafter, the tube is selectively opened for symptoms of gastric distention (nausea, vomiting, and bloating). None of the patients in their series needed to use the gastrostomy tube for gastric decompression beyond 24 hours postoperatively [18].

## 7. Conclusion

The diagnosis of gastric volvulus requires familiarity with the presenting signs and symptoms. Early diagnosis is critical to timely intervention. Surgeon experience and patient physiology will drive the surgical approach.

## Acknowledgements

This work was supported by the Department of Surgery at the University of Miami, Miller School of Medicine.

## Conflict of interest

The authors declare no conflict of interest.

## Author details

Maria Carolina Jimenez, Jose M. Martinez and Robert F. Cubas*
Department of Surgery, Miller School of Medicine, Jackson Health System, University of Miami, Miami, FL, USA

*Address all correspondence to: rcubas@miami.edu

## References

[1] Morelli U, Bravetti M, Ronca P, Cirocchi R, De Sol A, Spizzirri A, et al. Laparoscopic anterior gastropexy for chronic recurrent gastric volvulus: A case report. Journal of Medical Case Reports. 2008;**2**:244

[2] El Mouhafid FYM, Bounaim A, Moujahid M. Gastric volvulus: A challenge to diagnosis and management. World Journal of Surgery and Surgical Research. 2020;**3**:1236

[3] Imperatore K, Olivieri B, Vincentelli C. Acute gastric volvulus: A deadly but commonly forgotten complication of hiatal hernia. Autopsy & Case Reports. 2016;**6**(1):21-26

[4] Mazaheri P, Ballard DH, Neal KA, Raptis DA, Shetty AS, Raptis CA, et al. CT of gastric volvulus: Interobserver reliability, Radiologists' accuracy, and imaging findings. American Journal of Roentgenology. 2019;**212**(1):103-108

[5] Rashid F, Thangarajah T, Mulvey D, Larvin M, Iftikhar SY. A review article on gastric volvulus: A challenge to diagnosis and management. International Journal of Surgery. 2010;**8**(1):18-24

[6] Pandey S, Paudel M, Parajuli A, Ghimire R, Neupane A. Mesenteroaxial Gastric Volvulus: A Case Report. JNMA; Journal of the Nepal Medical Association. 2021;**59**(237):506-509

[7] Katkhouda N, Mavor E, Achanta K, Friedlander MH, Grant SW, Essani R, et al. Laparoscopic repair of chronic intrathoracic gastric volvulus. Surgery. 2000;**128**(5):784-790

[8] Naim HJ, Smith R, Gorecki PJ. Emergent laparoscopic reduction of acute gastric volvulus with anterior gastropexy. Surgical Laparoscopy, Endoscopy & Percutaneous Techniques. 2003;**13**(6):389-391

[9] Mistry V, Gamble EL, Chang J. Adult mesentero-axial gastric volvulus: Case report. Journal of Medical Imaging and Radiation Oncology. 2020;**64**(6):817-820

[10] Chau B, Dufel S. Gastric volvulus. Emergency Medicine Journal. 2007;**24**(6):446-447

[11] Kaoukabi AE, Menfaa M, Hasbi S, Sakit F, Choho A. Acute gastric volvulus on hiatal hernia. Case Rep Surg. 2020;**2020**:4141729

[12] Channer LT, Squires GT, Price PD. Laparoscopic repair of gastric volvulus. JSLS. 2000;**4**:225-230

[13] Light D, Links D, Griffin M. The threatened stomach: Management of the acute gastric volvulus. Surgical Endoscopy. 2016;**30**(5):1847-1852

[14] Coleman C, Musgrove K, Bardes J, Dhamija A, Buenaventura P, Abbas G, et al. Incarcerated paraesophageal hernia and gastric volvulus: Management options for the acute care surgeon, an eastern Association for the Surgery of trauma master class video presentation. Journal of Trauma and Acute Care Surgery. 2020;**88**(6):e146-e1e8

[15] Albloushi D, Quttaineh D, Alsafran S, Alyatama K, Alfawaz AA, Alsulaimy M, et al. Acute gastric volvulus: A rare case report and literature review. Ann Med Surg (Lond). 2021;**70**:102857

[16] Inaba K, Sakurai Y, Isogaki J, Komori Y, Uyama I. Laparoscopic repair of hiatal hernia with mesenterioaxial

volvulus of the stomach. World Journal of Gastroenterology. 2011;**17**(15): 2054-2057

[17] Teague WJ, Ackroyd R, Watson DI, Devitt PG. Changing patterns in the management of gastric volvulus over 14 years. The British Journal of Surgery. 2000;**87**(3):358-361

[18] Yates RB, Hinojosa MW, Wright AS, Pellegrini CA, Oelschlager BK. Laparoscopic gastropexy relieves symptoms of obstructed gastric volvulus in highoperative risk patients. American Journal of Surgery. 2015;**209**(5):875-880. discussion 80

[19] Martinez-Perez A, Garrigos-Ortega G, Gomez-Abril SA, Torres-Sanchez T, Uceda-Navarro D. Perforated gastric volvulus due to incarcerated paraesophageal hernia. Revista de Gastroenterología de México. 2014;**79**(3):204-206

[20] Pearson FG, Cooper JD, Ilves R, Todd TR, Jamieson WR. Massive hiatal hernia with incarceration: A report of 53 cases. The Annals of Thoracic Surgery. 1983;**35**(1):45-51

[21] Tartaglia N, Pavone G, Di Lascia A, Vovola F, Maddalena F, Fersini A, et al. Robotic voluminous paraesophageal hernia repair: A case report and review of the literature. Journal of Medical Case Reports. 2020;**14**(1):25

[22] Konstantinidis K, Konstantinidis M, Hirides SHP. Robotic hiatal hernia repair. In: Küçük S, editor. Surgical Robotics. London: IntechOpen; 2017. DOI: 10.5772/intechopen.71164

[23] Deugarte DA, Hirschl RB, Geiger JD. Robotic repair of congenital Paraesophageal hiatal hernia. Journal of Laparoendoscopic & Advanced Surgical Techniques. 2009;**19**(s1):s187-s1s9

[24] Aslam S, Alani M, Ansari Z, Moussa J, Srinivasan I, Chuang K-Y. S3156 gastric volvulus: An underrated complication of hiatal hernia. Official journal of the American College of Gastroenterology ACG. 2021;**116**:S1301

[25] Jindal S, Hukkeri VS, Qaleem M, Tandon V, Govil D. Robotic repair of a parahiatal hernia with gastric volvulus. Apollo Medicine. 2016;**13**(4):235-238

Section 3

# Malignant Diseases

Chapter 6

# Salvage Esophagectomy in Advanced Esophageal Cancer

*José Luis Braga de Aquino and Vânia Aparecida Leandro-Merhi*

## Abstract

Even through the esophageal cancer has innumerable treatment options, its prognosis is still unsettled. Because esophagectomy is rarely curative, others therapies, such as chemoradiation emerging in advanced disease followed or not surgery. The salvage esophagectomy is an alternative for those patients with recurrent disease. Thus in this chapter the intend is show the results of the salvage esophagectomy in patients with esophageal cancer who had previously undergone chemoradiation and discussion about the morbidity of this surgical tecnic. Too, its show the our experience in 72 patients with unresectabeled esophageal carcinoma were treated with chemorradiation followed by salvage esophagectomy by trans-toracic approach. Patients was evaluated with regard pos-operative complications and disease free survival. The major complications was deiscence at the level of the of the anastomosis esophagogastric cervical, presents in 16 patients (22,2%) and pulmonar infection in 23 patients (31,9%). In 53 patients that were available for a five years follow-up, was a rate of 43,3% (23 patients) of disease free survival. Thus with the results its conclude that the salvage esophagectomy seems to be valuable in cases without any other therapeutic options.

**Keywords:** salvage esophagectomy, esophageal neoplasms, esophagectomy, neoadjuvant, therapy, post-operative complications, quimioradiation

## 1. Introduction

Esophageal malignancy is still a rather frequent condition, ranking third among the most frequent tumors of the gastrointestinal tract and the eighth most prevalent in the world [1–4]. Recent studies show that esophagus neoplasms have increased by 10% per year, causing approximately 400,000 annual deaths and being the sixth leading cause of cancer death [5–7].

In Brazil, it is the seventh most common malignant neoplasm with an estimated 13,550 new cases in 2016; its highest incidence occurs in the South and Southeast regions of Brazil [8, 9].

The delay in diagnosis, excessive weight loss due to dysphagia and the association of cardiopulmonary diseases resulting from tobacco abuse make patients with a condition difficult to be controlled clinically, leaving their physicians with few therapeutic options [3, 4, 10, 11].

This reflects in the indication of esophagectomy. Although this surgical procedure remains to this day the best indication of therapy for a potential cure, because of the advanced stage of the disease found in most cases and also because of the great clinical nutritional depletion that affect patients, only 30 to 40% of them can undergo this treatment. This means that this condition has a rather unfavorable prognosis [1, 5, 11–13].

And even in patients who have clinical conditions that allow radical surgery, the prognosis is also rather poor; in fact, those patients have an average survival rate of only 15.5 months, with a two-year survival rate varying from 34 to 37% and with locoregional failure of up to 42%, as has been demonstrated in several recent studies [3, 5, 6, 10, 13, 14].

Thus, due to the low effectiveness of esophagectomy as a single treatment used with a curative purpose, for some years now new therapeutic measures have been advocated, such as radiotherapy and chemotherapy alone or associated in the pre- or post-operative period of surgical resection [5, 6, 12, 13, 15].

With the evolution of oncological therapy using more potent drug associations with fewer side effects and the advent of devices with better resolution and with more adequate techniques for performing radiotherapy, in recent years chemoradiation with exclusive intent has been suggested for a definite treatment for patients with locally advanced and unresectable esophageal cancer or patients without clinical and nutritional conditions for esophagectomy [3, 4, 6, 7, 16, 17].

However, studies with longer follow-up have shown that exclusive chemoradiation as a definitive therapy has also an unfavorable prognosis in advanced stage esophageal tumors, even if it is only with locoregional involvement without distant metastasis, with a median survival of 29 months, with local recurrence of up to 60% and a five-year survival ranging from 10 to 26% [1, 2, 4–6, 17].

Thus, the only way to attempt a potential cure in these patients with recurrence or persistence of the disease, after failure of exclusive chemoradiotherapy, would be salvage esophagectomy with a 5-year survival rate ranging from 25 to 40% [3, 4, 10, 11, 13, 16, 18].

Unlike planned esophagectomy, which is a full part of multimodal therapy for esophageal cancer, salvage esophagectomy is selectively indicated after chemoradiation failure as a definitive proposal [2, 3, 4, 6, 11, 16, 17]. In planned esophagectomy, after neoadjuvant chemoradiation, the surgical procedure is always performed, unless there is a contraindication for its performance, such as malignant disease progression or greater impairment of the patient's general condition [16–20].

However, the decision to perform salvage esophagectomy is often debatable, as it is often difficult to prove the persistence or recurrence of the disease. This is because, although patients may have clinical and imaging findings suggestive of malignancy, such as recurrent dysphagia and esophageal wall thickening, respectively, endoscopic biopsies are often inconclusive, due to persistent fibrosis from previous treatment.

If in the esophagectomy planned in the multimodal treatment, where the absence of tumor in the surgical specimen is considered a success, the finding of benign disease in the salvage esophagectomy can be considered a failure [2, 3, 19–21]. This is because salvage esophagectomy is another selective method of treatment in patients who still have persistent or recurrent locoregional tumors after chemoradiation failure [5, 7, 11, 21, 22]. Evidently, there are clinical situations in which the severity of the esophageal pathology justifies resection, even if it is a benign pathology, such as endoscopic intractable stenosis, ulcers and fistulas resulting from radiotherapy [3, 4, 20, 23].

Esophagectomy after chemoradiation, whether planned or salvage, can be technically difficult, since the radiation affects the mediastinum structures, either earlier, due to the presence of an inflammatory process, or later, due to the evolution to fibrosis [3, 12, 13, 22].

The greater tissue injury is caused by the highest irradiation dose, whether total or fractional, the greater extension of the irradiation field, and this may influence the greater morbidity of salvage esophagectomy [1, 4, 11, 19–21]. Some series have shown that tissue damage is greater in patients undergoing this type of resection, since the total dose used in chemoradiation with final intention is generally higher, and on average 50 to 60 Gy, for 30 to 40 Gy for the group of patients initially submitted to neoadjuvant therapy [12, 14, 24–26].

Another relevant fact is that in planned esophagectomy the time interval between the end of chemoradiation and the surgery is shorter (20 to 30 days), which means that there is still only an inflammatory process at the mediastinal level, whereas in salvage esophagectomy, because the interval for surgery is longer, on average, from 3 to 6 months, severe fibrosis develops, with increasing difficulty to dissect the esophagus with the mediastinal structures predisposing to a greater potential for morbidity [1, 15, 18, 22].

This fact, associated with skepticism regarding the cure for esophageal cancer, explains the reluctance of many surgeons to perform this type of procedure, because despite this therapeutic modality being more popular in recent years, some series have not yet demonstrated adequate standardization. This may hinder the results of the actual validity of salvage esophagectomy after previous chemoradiation with exclusive intent [15, 27–29].

In recent years, with the improved evolution and standardization of the surgical techniques, better assessment of postoperative complications, better standardization of staging by the latest TNM consensus [30], with a more adequate selection of patients with study variables that can be standardized in the same way, caused several series to begin showing better results with the use of salvage esophagectomy [3, 4, 6, 11, 13, 17, 19, 25].

## 2. Surgical procedure

### 2.1 Patients selection

A careful selection of patients is required, since in most cases they present with pulmonary involvement, as they have chronic obstructive pulmonary disease, in addition to the nutritional deficit worsened by previous chemoradiation.

Hence the importance of an adequate preoperative clinical evaluation with pulmonary function tests in which the expiratory volume of the first second (FEV1) and the pulmonary diffusing capacity (DLCO) are 50% greater than expected [18, 21].

Also in order to have a more adequate selection of patients, it would be desirable that they were non – smokers or having quit smoking at least 3 months prior to the surgery, and also underwent chest physiotherapy at least 30 days prior to the surgery [21, 31].

Regarding nutrition, it is important that patients perform a well-appropriate preoperative nutritional assessment, since most of these patients have marked nutritional deficits resulting not only from the chemotherapeutic treatment but also from the disease that may still be present or relapse. Thus, in recent years, some important indicators have been advocated for the assessment of the nutritional status:

a. Nutritional Risk Screening 2002 (NRS 20020): it is a nutritional screening instrument for determining nutritional risk, taking into account weight loss, reduced food consumption, body mass index and disease severity [32].

b. Subjective Global Assessment (SGA): is an instrument that subjectively assesses the nutritional status of the sick individual, based on scores given to weight loss, food consumption and clinical and physical signs of malnutrition [33].

c. Anthropometry indicators: the most common indicators are body weight, body mass index (BMI), arm circumference (AC), triceps skinfold (tsf), arm muscle circumference (AMC) and calf circumference (CC) [32–34].

d. Laboratory tests: tests associated with nutritional status, such as albumin, pre-albumin, transferrin and lymphocyte count.

After this evaluation, if it is confirmed that the patients are malnourished, parenteral or enteral nutrition is indicated during a variable time of 15 to 30 days in the preoperative period, depending on the degree of malnutrition.

## 2.2 Anesthetic act

Due to the fibrosis that occurs at the thoracic level, upon previous chemoradiation, it is recommended that the thoracic route be used, either by thoracotomy or videothoracoscopy to have easier access to the esophagus [3, 4, 35–37].

Thus, it is necessary to perform anesthesia with single-lung ventilation with a minimum fraction of inspired oxygen, to prevent further damage to the lung parenchyma, which is often already compromised by actinic action [11, 18, 31].

## 2.3 Surgical technique

### *2.3.1 Resection*

Despite the main objective of the surgery being the performance of a complete resection (R0), especially when this procedure is the primary treatment of cancer; this same strategy has to be applied carefully after chemoradiation. Thus, the salvage esophagectomy series indicate, in most cases, a resection of the entire thoracic esophagus until reaching the cervicothoracic transition, through direct vision, by right thoracotomy, to facilitate the dissection of the organ due to the presence of fibrosis that ensued previous radiotherapy and, therefore, minimizing complications [2, 4, 12, 13, 17, 20, 29].

In recent years with the advent of minimally invasive surgery, demonstrating the advantages of minor trauma, some series have proposed this access route. Ishiyama et al. [35], in a recent study, comparing salvage esophagectomy by videothoracoscopy in 20 patients against 62 patients submitted to this procedure using right thoracotomy, showed that there was a significantly lower incidence of pneumonia in the video group (20.0%) compared to the open surgery group (48.3%). According to these authors, this result is due to the fact that the prone position used in videothoracoscopy improves oxygenation when compared with thoracotomy, and artificial pneumothorax where the gravity condition when accessing the operative field induces less lung compression when compared with the right lateral decubitus position, thus resulting in less damage to the lung tissues, with concomitant reduction in atelectasis with preservation of oxygenation and, potentially, preventing postoperative pneumonia. This fact has also been demonstrated by other authors [36–38].

Recently, high-definition video systems for laparoscopic and thoracoscopic surgery have shown advantages over conventional open surgery, as they provide sharper images of the anatomical structure, which can often be quite distorted by previous radiotherapy [35, 38, 39]. Thus, the recognition of microanatomy is better recognized, with better preservation of nerves and vessels when compared to open surgery, thus being able to reduce blood loss [36, 37]. In addition this preservation of vessels is also important, especially in relation to the trachea wall, which is supplied by a network of vessels along its longitudinal face, and thus, with a better visualization of this anatomy, it is possible to prevent this organ ischemia with reduction of pneumonia and postoperative tracheal fistula [35, 39].

Regarding lymphadenectomy, there is no well-defined consensus, since some authors suggest routine lymph node dissection in II and III surgical fields and other authors only in lymph node stations with suspected metastases, to avoid devascularization of the airways [11, 19, 20, 29, 31, 35, 40].

Although there is controversy regarding the increase in overall survival, some authors have recently suggested salvage lymphadenectomy, that is, only lymphadenectomy, without esophageal resection, because the disease is only located in the locoregional lymph nodes, after chemoradiation with definitive intent, as it is less invasive and has a low incidence of complications [13, 41, 42]. Katoe et al. [41] demonstrated in 30 patients submitted to salvage lymphadenectomy that the overall survival was significantly higher when there was recurrence of the disease in the lymph nodes in relation to the residual disease in the same lymph nodes, being 21.7% to 0.0%, respectively; they also showed that overall survival was significantly higher when lymphadenectomy was performed outside the irradiation field, with 47.6% to 8.9%, of the patients, respectively.

Some authors have also advocated partial parietal pleurectomy during salvage esophagectomy, in order to promote a pleural symphysis and provide a more conservative conduct in the event of a potential lymphatic fistula [3, 29, 43].

#### 2.3.2 Esophageal reconstruction

Esophageal reconstruction, unlike the esophagectomy resection time, is responsible for most septic and pulmonary complications after surgery, which makes some authors recommend that it be performed in a second surgical procedure, especially in more nutritionally undermined patients and when the viscera to be transposed already presents a jeopardized perfusion [5, 27, 29, 43–45]. Although the organ to be transposed in the reconstruction may present a good perfusion in the abdomen, perfusion can be hindered by the anatomical distortion of the immediate transposition [14, 29, 43, 44].

Thus, some surgeons have supported reconstruction by gastric transposition to the cervical region 4 to 6 weeks after resection, although more recently other surgeons indicate their preference for a prompt reconstruction [2, 3, 5, 11, 13, 17, 29, 44, 45].

Although it is already well standardized that the reconstruction route is carried out through the posterior mediastinum because it is more anatomical and physiological, some authors still believe that the anterior mediastinal route is more favorable, as it minimizes the consequences of a probable anastomotic fistula at the cervical level besides being more easily diagnosed and managed. Most of the time drainage of the cervical region at bedside will do [3, 6, 7, 12, 18, 29, 44, 45].

A variant that has been proposed, although with little acceptance, in the framework of gastric transposition through the anterior mediastinal route is not performing an immediate esophagogastric anastomosis, with the advantage of minimizing the anastomotic fistula and aspiration of gastric contents into the airways [11, 23, 39, 43]. In addition, this access route has the advantage of avoiding tracheobronchial compression and preventing a fistula of the organ transposed with the airways.

## 3. Post-operative complications

With the evolution of chemoradiation, with greater potential as a definitive treatment for esophageal cancer, many series began to indicate salvage esophagectomy more frequently, especially in patients with recurrent tumors and with a stage less than or equal to T2 after oncological treatment [1, 2, 4, 11, 13, 14, 16, 20, 21].

Thus, it is important to remember the complications that this type of resection can cause, with a frequency of up to two or three times greater than that of esophagectomy without previous treatment [13, 15, 22, 29, 31]. Recently Mitchell et al. [18], comparing the postoperative morbidity of 35 patients undergoing salvage esophagectomy with 41 patients undergoing planned esophagectomy, showed complications with higher morbidity of 71.4% and 36.6%, respectively; and in the same comparison, mortality at 90 days after surgery was 17.1% and 9.8%, respectively.

Thus, the postoperative period of salvage esophagectomy is notable for several complications, especially those described below:

### 3.1 Respiratory failure

Although this complication does not fit a precise classification, adult respiratory distress syndrome and pneumonia are the two most frequent conditions [18, 21, 29, 46]. Chemoradiation, even without surgery, can already cause the respiratory distress syndrome and, associated with the surgical trauma of esophagectomy, predisposes more intensely to this syndrome [7, 12, 14].

Actinic pneumonia resulting from irradiation is probably the first injury to the lungs, and the release of cytokines during the surgical procedure would increase the intensity of the lung parenchyma injury [3, 18, 29, 46].

Mechanical ventilation during surgery or in the immediate postoperative period can also initiate an inflammatory cascade in the lungs, especially when there is a need for prolonged periods and single-lung ventilation with a high volume of the fraction of inspired oxygen, in addition to the perfusion in only one lung [46].

Lymphatic obstruction resulting from irradiation or surgical excision, for those authors who advocate mediastinal lymph node drainage, may also contribute to acute lung injury [19, 47].

Another well-known etiology, which can exacerbate the inflammatory cascade characteristic of adult respiratory distress syndrome, would be tissue ischemia with the stomach transposed for transit reconstruction, even if this is not sufficient to cause gastric necrosis [21, 23, 29].

Pneumonia after salvage esophagectomy has also many causes, such as chronic obstructive pulmonary disease, resulting from long-term smoking, present in most of these patients, is the most relevant factor, as has been demonstrated in several series [11, 13, 15, 20, 23, 27–29]. And this complication is also significantly lower in planned esophagectomy when compared to salvage esophagectomy, due to the lower intensity of irradiation in patients who undergo this type of surgical tactic after neoadjuvant chemoradiation [18, 21]. This was well demonstrated by Mitchell et al. [18] who, comparing 41 patients undergoing neoadjuvant therapy and planned esophagectomy with 35 patients undergoing salvage resection after chemoradiation with exclusive intent for having in the initial stage T4b presented an incidence of pneumonia from 12.2% to 34.3%, respectively. Hence it is important to perform a good preoperative preparation with adequate respiratory physiotherapy.

Also the great importance of the advent of video thoracoscopic surgery that offers the access route used for esophageal resection, potentially reduces the damage to lung tissue with reduced atelectasis and greater oxygenation and, consequently, a lower incidence of pulmonary infection, as has been recently demonstrated in some series [35, 37, 38].

The deficient nutritional status, characteristic in most patients with esophageal cancer, can be further exacerbated by previous chemoradiation which, associated with immunosuppression also present in those patients, can more often predispose to pneumonia. Hence it is important to perform an assessment and provide an adequate preoperative nutritional support, to try to minimize this complication.

Another fact that can also predispose to pulmonary infection is the edema of the cervical region resulting from the dissection of the esophagus which occurs in the first postoperative days and can hamper swallowing in a transient way and thus predispose to aspiration of secretions from the mouth cavity and pharynx into the tracheobronchial tree [29].

The introduction of a nasogastric tube to decompress the stomach in the immediate postoperative period also favors the release of the upper and lower esophageal sphincters and thus may cause reflux into the airways, with consequent pulmonary injury [29, 32].

### 3.2 Esophago-visceral anastomosis dehiscence

The etiology of esophagogastric anastomosis dehiscence is multifactorial, but technical errors and insufficient tissue perfusion of the gastric wall are the most important causes [31, 43]. Vascularization of the transposed stomach for esophageal reconstruction is performed by the right gastroepiploic and right gastric vessels, since the left gastric, left gastroepiploic and short vessels are sectioned. Thus the gastric duct survives because the stomach has a rich submucosal vascular plexus. Previous irradiation, especially with a dose > or equal to 50 Gy, can hamper the microcirculation of the gastric conduit, with consequent areas of necrosis and providing anastomotic dehiscence [21, 22, 29]. This was very evident in the review carried out by Jamel & Markar [21] who, in the evaluation of 11 studies with 1906 patients with esophageal cancer, showed that the group of patients undergoing salvage esophagectomy had significantly 21.8% anastomotic dehiscence for 8.1% of this complication for the group of patients undergoing planned esophagectomy. And this fact is also demonstrated by other authors [18, 28, 29, 31].

With the advent of mechanical sutures to perform anastomoses of the digestive tract, whether in benign or malignant conditions, perhaps this complication could be minimized in patients undergoing salvage esophagectomy. This is because this suture provides a better coaptation of the anastomotic stumps as it is double and inverted [48, 49].

The morbidity of esophageal-gastric anastomosis dehiscence depends on the location, whether cervical or thoracic, on the viability of the gastric conduit and on the conditions of the perianastomotic tissues, to try to block the fistula resulting from the dehiscence. The most favorable situation is when dehiscence occurs in the cervical region with a viable gastric conduit and protected by the soft tissues around the anastomosis.

The management for the treatment of this complication is based on the severity of the dehiscence. If severe, early and in the thoracic region and with hemodynamic undermining, aggressive surgical intervention is mandatory; however, if this complication occurs later, usually after the fifth postoperative day and in the cervical region, the conduct may be more conservative, with drainage of the cervical region at the bedside [43, 45, 48, 49]. However, conservative management of this complication after salvage esophagectomy can often be unsuccessful if the tissue bed at the level of the anastomosis has been irradiated [18, 21, 29].

### 3.3 Recurrent laryngeal nerve injury

Recurrent laryngeal nerve injury can occur in any esophagectomy technique, but this complication is more common after salvage esophagectomy due to mediastinal fibrosis resulting from irradiation, which causes intense adhesions of this nerve to the esophagus and to the mediastinal lymph nodes, making dissection difficult [3, 5, 10, 11, 22, 31].

As a consequence, this lesion causes vocal cord paralysis, a complication that is poorly tolerated by patients undergoing salvage esophagectomy, as it promotes pulmonary aspiration more frequently, limits the patient's ability to cough and thus worsens already existing lung lesions due to actinic action.

### 3.4 Airway necrosis

Extensive necrosis of the trachea is a rare but usually fatal complication after salvage esophagectomy [19, 29, 43]. On the other hand, focal necrosis of the airways is more common, with a rate of up to 23%, in most series that demonstrate this type of complication [4, 24, 43, 50].

And this complication may occur due to mediastinal fibrosis resulting from previous more intense irradiation, which predisposes to inadvertent injuries to the airways during the surgical procedure that, associated with vascular damage resulting from actinic obliterating endarteritis can induce airway necrosis. This complication has caused some authors to avoid the large dissections of three-field esophagectomy, as this procedure is more indicated in esophagectomy without previous chemoradition to minimize those complications [12, 15, 17–19, 24].

This complication, once present, is evidenced by a fistula in the mediastinum and/or pleura, progressing to pneumomediastinum or pneumothorax.

Conservative treatment of these fistulas is controversial, since, due to previous irradiation, the tissue injury at the mediastinal level becomes difficult to be blocked. And this treatment becomes even more difficult when the necrotic segment of the tracheobronchial tree develops a fistula into the stomach transposed to the posterior mediastinum, since, besides having difficulty in ventilation, a continuous aspiration of gastric secretion into the lungs occurs [29, 43, 50]. Although treatment with a self-expanding prosthesis is a valid option, it can, though, worsen the airway ischemia [43].

### 3.5 Chylothorax

This is a complication that, although quite uncommon, can also occur due to the difficulty in identifying the thoracic duct during esophageal dissection, resulting from intense mediastinal fibrosis caused by previous irradiation [29, 31]. Mitchell et al. [18], comparing the incidence of this complication among patients undergoing planned and salvage esophagectomy, showed that this complication was null for 11.4% in both cases. Lymphatic fistulas with high output, generally exceeding 1 liter per day, has early surgical indication, with thoracic duct ligation [18, 29]. On the other hand, with low-output fistulas, the conduct may be conservative, associating parenteral nutrition, chest drainage, and chemical pleurodesis [18, 29, 31].

## 4. Post-surgical care

Sepsis is the leading cause of mortality after salvage esophagectomy. It often starts with pulmonary involvement and ends with multiple-organ failure.

Thus, to prevent this morbid sequence, the surgical team must detect septic complications as early as possible and initiate aggressive treatment. Time is often lost in the evolution of the patient's septic condition when it is thought that the infection is a consequence of pulmonary atelectasis or urinary tract infection. Gastric necrosis and anastomotic dehiscence, especially if it occurs up to the third postoperative day as well as pleural empyema and intraperitoneal abscess are important septic complications to consider [18, 22, 23, 28, 46].

Hence the importance of performing upper digestive endoscopy as early as possible when gastric necrosis is suspected, which, if confirmed, has an immediate indication for a new surgery with resection of the interposed stomach [18, 29]. If there is clinical evidence of a fistula with secretion drainage through the incision in the cervical region and without hemodynamic repercussions, drainage of this region should be performed through cervicotomy at bedside [23, 29, 43, 45].

Patients undergoing salvage resection, because their general condition is more undermined, require the most adequate nutritional support. Thus, in addition to an adequate intermittent nutritional assessment in the postoperative period, it is also of fundamental importance to carry out a careful investigation of short- and long-term food intake after esophageal resections. This is because the changes that may occur in the process of nutrient absorption as a result of the surgical procedure performed, cause many patients, even six months after surgery, to be unable to meet their energy, protein and micronutrient requirements [51–53].

Hence, some researchers suggest the supplementation of the oral diet with an enteral diet, even in the postoperative period, in the medium term after esophageal resection [51, 54, 55].

## 5. Survival

More recently, some series have shown that the results, in terms of medium and long-term survival after salvage esophagectomy, are better in patients with residual or recurrent tumor classified as T2 or less after chemoradiation with previously definitive intent and also R0 resection [6, 7, 11, 13, 17, 21, 56].

This was well demonstrated in the study by Okamura et al. [17] who, evaluating 35 patients who underwent salvage esophagectomy after chemoradiation with exclusive intent, had 2 and 5-year survival rates with T2 tumors, of 85% and 65%, respectively; 20% and 0% survival, respectively with tumors greater than or equal to T3; and the same in relation to resection, since at 2 and 5 years there was 50% and 33% survival with R0 resection and 15% and 0% with resection R1/R2.

Fujita et al. [57] also demonstrated in a prospective, non-randomized study, in 53 patients, the need for esophagectomy after exclusive radical chemoradiation. In patients who did not fully respond to chemoradiation, surgical resection increased survival from 3 to 5 years, with a rate of 38% and 27%, respectively, and in most of these patients with T2 tumors the resection was R0.

Hence, it is important to proceed with an adequate patients' selection in the preoperative period, using well-suited imaging exams to assess the tumor extension. Of course, this can be difficult, because of the anatomical changes that occur due to the previous treatment that causes thickening of the esophageal wall.

Okamura et al. [17], evaluating this variable, demonstrated in their series that there was an accuracy of 91.4% with the use of high-resolution chest tomography between the pre and postoperative periods, in relation to the thickness of the tumor. However they suggest that, if there is any doubt about this information, PET-CT and echoendoscopy are indicated.

More recently, it has been demonstrated that the complications that may occur in the immediate postoperative period could have an impact on the survival of patients, due to the deterioration of the general and nutritional status causing an immunity deficit [11, 31]. In addition, postoperative complications can cause prolonged inflammation and produce inflammatory cytokines, which can induce tumor cell proliferation [11, 58].

This was clearly evidenced in the study by Sugimura et al. [31] who, assessing 73 patients who underwent salvage esophagectomy, showed that the 3- and 5-year overall survival of patients with some postoperative complication was 29.4% and 29.4% respectively, compared with 59.9% and 54.9%, respectively, among patients without any postoperative complications.

It is thus important to proceed with a good preoperative evaluation and careful monitoring in the intra and postoperative period to try to minimize this morbidity.

It has been shown that low albumin level, high C-reactive protein level, low body mass index, excessive intraoperative blood loss, poor nutritional status, advanced stage tumors and clinically positive lymph nodes and greater or equal irradiation at 60Gy, are variables associated with a higher occurrence of postoperative complications [11, 31].

## 6. Experience of the thoracic surgery service of hospital PUC-Campinas Brazil

From January 1995 to December 2021, 573 patients underwent esophagectomy for esophageal squamous cell carcinoma. Out of these, 72 underwent salvage esophagectomy for residual or recurrent disease after previous chemoradiation with exclusive intent and having an initial stage T4b.

At restagement for indication of salvage surgery, 59 patients (81.9%) had T2 or smaller tumors, and 13 (18.1%) T3/T4a.

All patients underwent esophageal resection by right thoracotomy and reconstruction of the digestive tract with gastric transposition to the cervical region in the first or second surgical procedure.

In the early postoperative evaluation regarding complications, 16 patients (22.2%) presented with cervical esophagogastric anastomosis dehiscence with good evolution fistula with conservative treatment in 15 patients; 3 patients (4.1%) had chylous fistula, and surgical treatment was indicated in 2 of them, with good evolution; 9 patients (12.5%) had recurrent laryngeal nerve paralysis, being definitive in 2 of them; 23 patients (31.9%) had pneumonia with good evolution, with specific treatment in 19 of them; 2 patients (2.7%) had a fatal cardiovascular event due to probable pulmonary thromboembolism.

Seven patients (9.7%) died due to complications in the first 30 days after surgery.

In the late evaluation, it was possible to follow up 53 patients for disease-free survival assessment: at 1 year – 51 patients (96.2%); at 3 years – 26 patients (49.0%) and at 5 years –23 (43.3%) patients. All patients who survived up to 5 years had T2 stage tumor or lower and underwent R0 resection.

## 7. Final considerations

Exclusive chemoradiotherapy in esophageal cancer has become quite popular in recent years, especially in cases with advanced locoregional disease and in those patients without physiological reserve for esophagectomy. With the evolution of nutritional support that was developed more recently, many patients were able to recover their general conditions, becoming fit for surgical resection.

In recent years, several series have demonstrated that salvage esophagectomy is technically feasible, despite the high morbidity, especially with regard to septic complications and adult respiratory distress syndrome. As these postoperative complications can infer a worse prognosis in the survival of these patients, it is important to prevent these complications and to keep these patients monitored for a long time in the postoperative period, especially with regard to nutritional status.

And this is important, because salvage esophagectomy is the only cure for cases of recurrence or persistence of the disease after exclusive chemoradiation. It therefore represents the best second-line treatment for local failure after exclusive chemoradiation, although further studies are needed to assess whether persistent disease has a worse prognosis than the recurrent disease after esophageal resection.

## Acknowledgements

To Hospital Puc-Campinas.

## Conflict of interest

The authors declare no conflict of interest.

## Author details

José Luis Braga de Aquino* and Vânia Aparecida Leandro-Merhi
Postgraduate Program of Health Sciences, Pontifical Catholic University of Campinas, Campinas, SP, Brazil

*Address all correspondence to: jlaquino@sigmanet.com.br

## References

[1] Kumagai K, Mariosa D, Tsai JÁ, Nilsson M, Ye W, Lundell L, et al. Systematic review and meta analysis on the significance of salvage esophagectomy for persistent or recurrent esophageal squamous cell carcinoma after chemoradiotherapy. Diseases of the Esophagus. 2016;**29**(7):734-739

[2] Swisher SG, Marks J, Rice D. Salvage esophagectomy for persistent or recurrent disease after definitive chemoradiation. Annals of Cardiothoracic Surgery. 2017;**6**(2):144-151

[3] Fajardo R, Abbas AE, Petrov RU, Bakhos CT. Salvage esophagectomy. The Surgical Clinics of North America. 2021;**101**(3):467-482

[4] Watanabe M. Salvage esophagectomy for residual tumor after definitive chemoradiotherapy for esophageal squamous cell carcinoma invading the neighboring organs. Is it a feasible choice? Annals of Surgical Oncology. 2020;**34**(5):123-129

[5] Sohda M, Kuwano H. Current status and future prospects for esophageal cancer treatment. Annals of Thoracic and Cardiovascular Surgery. 2017;**23**(1):1-11

[6] Watanabe M, Otake R, Kozuki R, Tochata T, Taka-Hashi K, Okamura A, et al. Recent progress in multidisciplinary treatment for patients with esophageal cancer. Surgery Today. 2020;**50**(1):12-20

[7] Swisher SG, Moughan J, Komaki RU, Ajani JA, Wu TT, Hofstetter WL, et al. Final results of NRG on oncology RTOG 0246: In organ-preserving selective resection strategy in esophageal cancer patient treated with definitive chemoradiation. Journal of Thoracic Oncology. 2017;**12**(1):368-374

[8] Instituto Nacional do Câncer. Incidência de câncer no Brasil: estimativa 2016. Rio de Janeiro: Inca; 2016. Disponível em: http://www.inca.gov.br/estimativa 2016. [Acesso: abril 23, 2017]. Portuguese

[9] Tustumi F, Kimura CMS, Takeda FR, Sallum RAA, Ribeiro Junior U, Ceconello I. Evaluation of lymphatic spread, visceral metastasis and tumoral local invasion in esophageal carcinomas. ABCD Arquivos Brasileiros de Cirurgia Digestiva. 2016;**29**(4):215-217. DOI: 10.1590/0102-672020 1600040001

[10] Yuan X, Jiahua LV, Dong H, Wang J. Does cervical lymphonode recurrence after oesophagectomy or definitive chemoradiotherapy for thoracic esophageal squamous cell carcinoma benefit from salvage treatment? Interactive Cardiovascular Thoracic Surgery. 2017;**27**(5):792-795

[11] Kiyozumi Y, Yoshida N, Ishimoto T, Yagi T, Koga Y, Uchihara T, et al. Prognostic factors of salvage esophagectomy for residual or recurrent esophageal squamous cell carcinoma after definitive chemoradiotherapy. World Journal of Surgery. 2018;**42**(9):2887-2893

[12] Lerbutsayanukul C, Tharavej C, Klaikea WN, Prayongrat A, Lowanitchai C, Sriuranpong V. High dose radiation with chemotherapy followed by salvage esophagectomy among patients with locally advanced esophageal squamous cell carcinoma. Thoracic Cancer. 2017;**8**(3):219-228

[13] Yagi K, Toriui T, Aikou S, Yamashita H, Seto Y. Salvage treatment after definitive chemoradiotherapy for

esophageal squamous cell carcinoma. Annals of Gastroenterological Surgery. 2021;**5**:436-445

[14] Farinella E, Safar A, Nasser H, Bouazza F, Libera-Lle G, Paesmans M, et al. Salvage esophagectomy after failure of definitive radiochemotherapy for esophageal cancer. Journal of Surgical Oncology. 2016;**114**(7):833-837

[15] Zhou N, Hofstteter WL, Esopahgeal Squamous Cell Carcinoma Working Group, Mitchell KG, Bayley EM, Ajani JA, et al. Salvage esophagectomy definition influences comparative outcomes in esophageal squamous cell cancers. The Annals of Thoracic Surgery. 2021;**29**:23-29

[16] Barbetta A, Hsu M, Tan KS. Definitive chemoradiotherapy versus neoadjuvant chemoradiotherapy followed by surgery for stage II to III esophageal squamous cell carcinoma. The Journal of Thoracic and Cardiovascular Surgery. 2018;**155**:2710-2721

[17] Okamura A, Hayami M, Kozuki R, Takahashi K, Toihata T, Imamura Y, et al. Salvage esophagectomy for initially unresectable locally advanced T4 esophageal squamous cell carcinoma. Esophagus. 2020;**17**:59-60

[18] Mitchell KG, Nelson DB, Corsini EM, Vaporciyan AA, Antonoff MB, Mehran RJ, et al. Morbidity following salvage esophagectomy for squamous cell carcinoma: The MD Anderson experience. Diseases of the Esophagus. 2020;**33**:3-doz067

[19] Ohkura Y, Ueno M, Iizuka T, Udagawa H. Prognostic factors and appropriate lymph node dissection in salvage esophagectomy for locally advanced T4 esophageal cancer. Annals of Surgical Oncology. 2019;**26**(1): 209-216

[20] Booka E, Haneda R, Ishi K, Kawakami T, Tsushima T, Yasui H, et al. Appropriate candidates for salvage esophagectomy of initially unresectable locally advanced T4 esophageal squamous cell carcinoma. Annals of Surgical Oncology. 2020;**27**(9):3163-3170

[21] Jamel S, Markar SR. Salvage esophagectomy: Safe therapeutic strategy? Journal of Thoracic Disease. 2017;**9**(8):799-808

[22] Low DE, Kuppusamy MK, Alderson D. Benchmarking complications associated with esophagectomy. Annals of Surgery. 2019;**269**(2):291-298

[23] Aquino JLB, Andreollo NA, Lopes LR. Terapêutica cirúrgica paliativa do câncer de esôfago. In: Fraga G, Aquino JLB, Andreollo NA. Atualidades em clinica cirúrgica. intergastro e trauma. Rio de Janeiro: Ed. Atheneu; 2010:283-294

[24] Kawakami T, Tsushima T, Omae K, Ogawa H, Shirasu H, Kito Y, et al. Risk factors for esophageal fistula in thoracic esophageal squamous cell carcinoma invading adjacent organs treated with definitive chemoradiotherapy: A monocentric case-control study. BMC Cancer. 2018;**18**(1):573-581

[25] Myata H, Sugmura K, Motoori M, Omori T, Yamamoto K, Yanagimoto Y. Clinical implications of conversion surgery after induction therapy for T4b thoracic esophageal squamous cell carcinoma. Annals of Surgical Oncology. 2019;**26**(13):4737-4743

[26] Saeki H, Tsutumi S, Tajiri H, Yukaya T, Tsutumi R, Nishimura S. Prognostic significance of post operative complications after curative resection for patients with esophageal squamous cell carcinoma. Annals of Surgery. 2017;**265**(3):527-533

[27] Markar S, Gronnier C, Duhamel A, Pasquer A, Théreaux J, du Rieu MC, et al. Salvage surgery after chemoradiotherapy in the management of esophageal cancer: Is it a viable therapeutic option? Journal of Clinical Oncology. 2015;**33**:3866-3873

[28] Pinto CE, Fernandes DS, Carvalho AL. Salvage esophagectomy after exclusive chemoradiotherapy: Results at the Brazilian National Cancer Institute (INCA). Diseases of the Esophagus. 2009;**22**:682-686

[29] Aquino JLB, Said MM, Pereira DAR, Cecchino GN, Leandro-Merhi VA. Complications of the rescue esophagectomy in advanced esophageal cancer. ABCD Arquivos Brasileirois de Cirurgia Digestiva. 2013;**26**(3):173-178

[30] Brierley JD, Gospodarowicz MK, Wittekind C. TNM Classification of Malignant Tumors: International Union Against Cancer. 8th ed. Oxford: Wiley; 2017

[31] Sugimura K, Myata H, Shinno N, Ushigome H, Asukai K, Hara H, et al. Prognostic impact of Postoperative complications following salvage esophagectomy for esophageal cancer after definitive chemoradiotherapy. Oncology. 2020;**98**(5):280-288

[32] Kondrup J, Rasmussen HH, Hamberg O, Stanga Z, ESPEN Working Group. Nutritional risk screening (NRS 2002): A new method based on a analysis of controlled clinical trials. Clinical Nutrition. 2003;**22**(3):321-336

[33] Dcnt E, Hoogendijk EO, Visvanathan R, Wright ORL. Malnutrition screening and assessment in hospitalized older people: A review. The Journal of Nutrition, Health & Aging. 2019;**23**(5):431-441

[34] Aquino JLB, Andreollo NA, Lopes LR. Esofagectomia de resgate no câncer de esôfago. In: Fraga GP, Pereira GS, Lopes LR, editors. Atualidades em clínica cirúrgica intergastro e trauma. 2a ed. Rio de Janeiro: Ed. Atheneu; 2011. pp. 307-318

[35] Ishiyama K, Oguma J, Kubo K, Kanematsu K, Kurita D, Daiko H. Salvage minimally invasive esophaagectomy after definitive chemoradiotherapy for esophageal câncer can improve postoperative complications compared with salvage open esophagectomy. Surgical Endoscopy. 2022;**36**(5):3504-3510

[36] Yoshida N, Yamamoto H, Baba H, Myyata H, Watanabe M, Toh Y, et al. Can minimally invasive esophagectomy replace open esophagectomy for esophageal cancer? Latest analysis of 24,233 esophagectomies from Japanese national clinical database. Annals of Surgery. 2020;**272**(1):118-124

[37] Defize IL, Van Der Horst S, Bulbul M, Mohammad NH, Mook S, Meijer GJ, et al. Salvage Robot-Assisted Minimally invasive esophagectomy (RAMIE) for T4b esophageal cancer after definitive chemoradiotherapy. Annals of Surgical Oncology. 2021;**28**(5):2730-2738

[38] Yamashita K, Mine S, Toihata T, Fukudome I, Okamura A, Yuda M, et al. The usefulness of three-dimensional video-assisted thorascoscopic esophagectomy in esophageal cancer patients. Esophagus. 2019;**16**(3):272-277

[39] Harada H, Kanaji S, Hasegawa H, Yamamoto M, Matsuda Y, Yamashita K, et al. The effect on surgical skills of expert surgeons using 3D/HD and 2D/K resolution monitors in laparoscopic phantom tasks. Surgical Endoscopy. 2018;**32**(10):4228-4234

[40] Sugawara K, Yagi K, Okumura Y, Nishida M, Aikou S, Yamashita H. Long term outcome of multimodal therapy combining definitive chemoradiotherapy and salvage surgery for T4 esophageal squamous cell carcinoma. International Journal of Clinical Oncology. 2020;**25**(4):552-560

[41] Kato F, Monma S, Koyanagi K, Kanamori J, Daiko H, Igaki H. Long term outcome after resection for recurrent oesophageal cancer. Journal of Thoracic Disease. 2018;**10**(5):2691-2699

[42] Yuan X, Lv J, Dong H, Wang J. Does cervical lymph node recurrence after oesophagectomy or definitive chemoradiotherapy for thoracic oesopahgeal squamous cell carcinoma benefit from salvage treatment? Interactive Cardiovascular and Thoracic Surgery. 2017;**24**(5):792-795

[43] Urschel JD, Sellke FW. Complications of salvage esophagectomy. Medical Science Monitor. 2003;**9**(7):173-180

[44] Stein HJ, Bartels H, Siewert JR. Esophageal carcinoma: 2-stage operation for preventing mediastinitis in high risk patients. Chirurg. 2001;**72**(8):881-886

[45] Urschel JD, Urschel DM, Miller JD, Bennett WF, Young JE. A meta-analysis of randomized controlled trials of route of reconsctruction after esohagectomy for cancer. American Journal of Surgery. 2001;**182**(5):470-475

[46] Tandon S, Batchelor A, Bullock R, Gascoigne A, Griffin M, Hayes N, et al. Periooperative risk factors for acute lung injury after eletive oesophagectomy. British Journal of Anaesthesia. 2001;**86**(5):633-638

[47] Cui Y, Urschell JD, Petrelli NJ. The effect of cardiopulmonar lymphatic obstruction on heart and lung function. The Journal of Thoracic and Cardiovascular Surgery. 2002;**49**:35-40

[48] Aquino JLB, Leandro-Merhi VA, Mendonça JÁ, Mendes EDT, Clairet CMAV, Reis LO. Comparative analysis of late results of cervical esophagogastric anastomosis by manual and mechanical suture in patients submitted to esophageal mucosectomy through advanced megaesophagus. ABCD Arquivos Brasileirois de Cirurgia Digestiva. 2019;**32**(4):1-5. DOI: 10.1590/0102-672020190001e1462

[49] Honda M, Kariyama A, Noma H, Nunobe S, Furkawa T. Hand-sewn versus mechanical esophagogastric anastomosis after esopahgectomy: A systematic review and meta-analysis. Annals of Surgery. 2013;**257**(2):238-248

[50] Bartels HE, Stein HJ, Siewert JR. Tracheobronquial lesions following oesohagectomy: Prevalence predisposing factors and outcome. The British Journal of Surgery. 1998;**85**(3):403-406

[51] Baker ML, Halliday V, Robinson P, Smith K, Bowrey DJ. Nutrient intake and contribution of home enteral nutrition to meeting nutritional requeriments after oesophagectomy and total gastrectomy. European Journal of Clinical Nutrition. 2017;**71**(9):1121-1128

[52] Haverkort EB, Binnekade JM, de Haan RJ, Busch OR, Van Berge Henegouwen MI, Gouma DJ. Suboptimal intake of nutrients after esophagectomy with gastric tube reconstruction. Journal of the Academy of Nutrition and Dietetics. 2021;**112**(7):1081-1087

[53] Leandro-Merhi VA, Aquino JLB, Reis LO. Predictors of nutritional risk according toNRS-2002 and calf circumference in hospitalized older adults with neoplasms. Nutrition and Cancer. 2017;**69**(8):1219-1226

[54] Ryan AM, Rowley HLA, Flood PM, Ravi N, Reynolds JV. Post-esophagectomy early enteral nutrition via a needle catheter jejunostomy: A 8-year experience at a specialist unit. Clinical Nutrition. 2006;**25**(3):386-393

[55] Leandro-Merhi VA. Braga de Aquino JL. Comparison of nutritional diagnosis methods and prediction of clinical outcomes in patients with neoplasms and digestive tract diseases. Clinical Nutrition. 2015;**34**(4):647-651

[56] Yokota T, Yasuda T, Kato H, Nozaki I, Sato H, Miyata Y, et al. Concordance of clinical diagnosis of T classification among physicians for locally advanced unresectable thoracic esophageal cancer. International Journal of Clinical Oncology. 2018;**23**(1):73-80

[57] Fujita H, Sueyoshi S, Tanaka T, Tanaka Y, Matono S, Mori N, et al. Esophagectomy: Is it necessary after chemoradiotherapy for a locally advanced T4 esophageal cancer? Prospective non randomized Trial comparing chemoradiotherapy with surgery versus without surgery. World Journal of Surgery. 2005;**29**(1):25-31

[58] Okamura A, Takeuchi H, Matsuda S. Factors affecting cytokine change after esophagectomy for esophageal cancer. Annals of Surgical Oncology. 2015;**22**(9):3130-3135